BROAD AXE TRAINING

Broad Axe Training:

A Frill-Free Approach to Strength & Conditioning

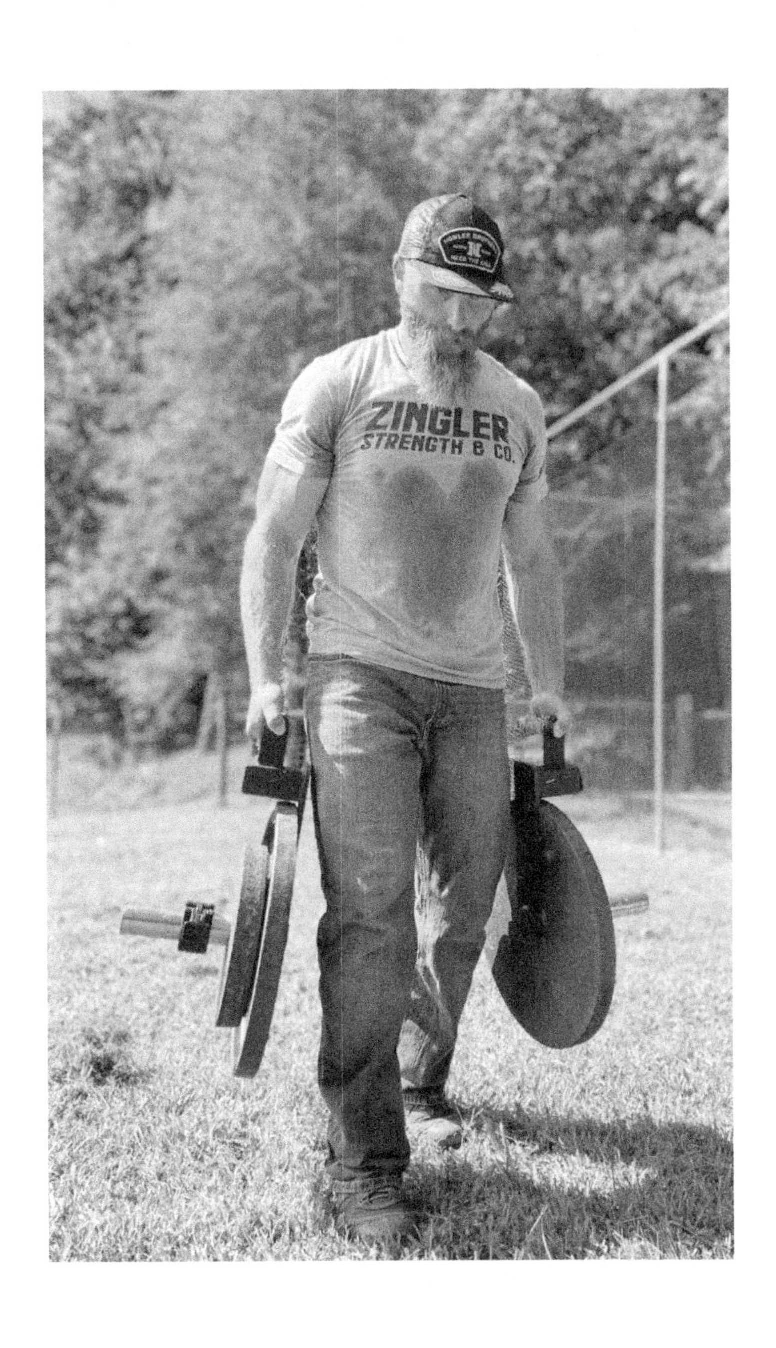

Disclaimer: Before embarking on any Physical Fitness Program, please consult your doctor, athletic trainer, or therapist.

Please recognize all exercise involves some inherent risk. If you are uncomfortable or unfamiliar with any exercise recommendations in this work, please seek counsel from a qualified professional.

Zingler Strength & Conditioning, LLC. and Ray Zingler disclaim any liability or loss in connection with the use of this program or any advice herein.

This book may not be reproduced or recorded in any form without permission from the author.

Copyright 2022 by Ray Zingler. All Rights Reserved

This work is dedicated to my family. Thank you for supporting me in my relentless, endless pursuit of serving others by way of my passion that is Strength & Conditioning.

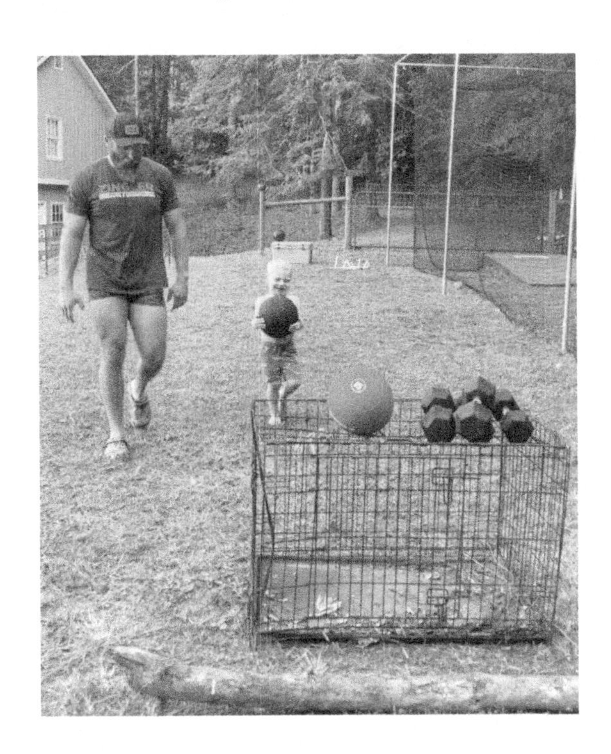

Table of Contents

Acknowledgments

This would not have been possible without the support of my family and those who have poured into me from near and far.

I can assure you, anything that works in this system is because of the intelligence of those with brighter minds than mine. Any errors in this system, I assure you are my own.

To Jim Wendler, Joe DeFranco, Dan John, Zach Even-Esh, Vernon Griffith, Pavel Tsatsouline, Joel Jamieson, Buddy Morris, Dave Tate, Louie Simmons (RIP), and many others, your impact and influence on my training and my life has been paramount. This system is a byproduct of my time spent studying & experimenting with your work. Keep living the code.

Thank you to all of my Zingler Strength & Conditioning Family, Social Media Supporters, and colleagues in the field.

It is because of you, I am full of an abundance of gratitude and have a rich desire to serve others.

Thank you for all the support.

Foreword

It is with great honor that I have been given the opportunity to write the foreword to Ray Zingler's first book. A book that will not only share his training lessons and methods, but more importantly, a book that will share his life lessons that his own kids and grandkids will eventually read. From afar, I get to see what Ray does in both his strength & conditioning as well as his life. And although these are just snippets, every video he shares on social tells a story; Put in the work, love your family and give nothing less than your best.

Ray and his athletes are hammering the basics. They are putting in the work. And although hard work on the basics sounds so simple, it's actually quite complicated. Many Coaches (young & veteran Coaches) and lifters / athletes screw this up, because they are seeking a way around the work. *What is the shortcut?* The answer is simple. The shortcut is through the work.

Training has gotten extremely fancy and too complicated. There is an overabundance of technology, and although there is merit to the technology, it will never and can never replace a Coach who genuinely cares for the athlete and takes the time to get under the bar himself / herself to learn through doing the work. Technology will not replace the life lessons you learn that come through good old-fashioned WORK.

Walk into any commercial gym today and it's a far cry from the type of gyms I grew up in and where I learned. No, this is not one of those *Back in the day* stories, this is the truth. This is about coming to terms with what works when it comes to training and the big missing link in today's training is a lack of .... WORK.

Heads are buried in phones. People will sit on a lat machine or lay down on a bench and *never get up,* because in between sets, they are on their phones. You'll never get strong that way. When you're training you must learn to become someone else. Your alter ego must kick in. You need to lose yourself and find yourself all at the same time. And that will never happen when you're busy scrolling through your phone, watching other people live their lives.

I grew up in the 80s, and so I believe I got lucky. I watched Rocky III the Summer before 3rd grade. I was with my older brother and as soon as Rocky ended, he took me out for a run. We ran with our Doberman which was like getting pulled by a horse. In today's fancy talk, we call that overspeed training. That's a joke of course, but I'm also partially serious. After the run, my brother had already collected some weights for his room, so we did curls and push ups. He didn't count sets, everything was done until we could no longer lift our arms. The next morning, I remember being unable to comb my hair and when I was about to call my Mom to tell her, my older brother threatened my life as he feared he would be grounded.

By the age of 8, I learned that push ups, curls and running were supposed to be normal activities. Today, we have high school football players unable to perform 1 push up. We have Coaches against running 400 meters let alone a mile if you play in power sports like Football and Baseball. Well, if you're a teenager, running a mile should *not be a problem.* You should be capable. So before you go searching for your favorite pro athlete workout on Instagram, go and watch Rocky III and Rocky IV.

That is the program you should follow; running through the hills, sprinting the streets, jumping over park benches, push ups, sit ups and squat jumps while holding a random tree log. This is the kind of "program" I had my athletes follow when I first began training athletes from my parents garage and backyard. Basketball players, wrestlers, baseball players and Football players were carrying stones in the backyard, doing pull ups off of tree branches with a towel draped over for grip strength, chopping wood, sprinting the hill that led up to the water towers and pushing my truck across empty parking lots.

I copied training from Rocky films and golden era bodybuilders of the 60s and 70s. Basic barbell training. The theme was hard work on the basics.

Everyone got bigger, faster and stronger. Athletes who struggled to make the team now made varsity and became leaders, not just in sports but in the way they communicated and behaved in and out of school.

Almost by accident, I knew we were onto something. It reminds me of two quotes I have heard through the years; *Simple things done savagely well,* and, *Brilliance with the basics.* Even to this day, with 25+ years of coaching and 33+ years of training, I catch myself getting away from the basics and I ask myself, *Is anyone here squatting 405? Benching 300?* Those were actually common numbers from my first location of The Underground Strength Gym. These athletes lifted hard and heavy, jumped high, ran fast and ate big. Afterwards they would play pick-up Basketball games at the local park, even the wrestlers played Basketball.

On their own, they ran hill sprints and did extra calisthenics. This was done in addition to mandatory school workouts and training at The Underground Strength Gym. Today, parents get scared that 1 or 2 training sessions in season will be too much for their son or daughter. They ask me, *Do you think this will be too much? I don't want him to get hurt!* The tone of voice sounds as if the world will end. I remind them, in the 80s, we played outside every weekend and all Summer long from 7 AM until 10 PM, only to come home for dinner. Nobody was "overtrained" from endless miles of bike riding or playing Basketball and Man Hunt for 4 hours a day.

The human body has amazing potential but if you plant the seeds of doubt, excuses, weakness and trying to make everything perfect, you will never get strong. NEVER. Sports, competition, and life are far from perfect. The body needs strength. Can you do 25 push-ups? 10 Pull Ups? Run a mile? If not, then stop worrying about "speed and agility" and start training like Rocky.

With "Strength Coaches" on every corner of almost every town, why do we have youth baseball players with fractured backs and broken elbows? Because parents fear strength yet they are OK with their kid swinging a bat at max effort from age 5 until age 15 with NO strength training. I can run down the list of other sports injuries but by now, hopefully you get the point.

It's time to build the body AND the mind. Train hard and train consistently. Wash it all down with a glass of whole milk and some steak and potatoes. Do this for YEARS. It's not a few weeks or months, if you truly want success, this is going to take years. And that right there is the beauty of it all because the Work is the Gift!

Live The Code 365,

Zach Even – Esh

PREFACE

Broad Axe Training: The System.

Broad Axe Training, where did that name come from?

My father, who is one of the greatest men I know, was a College Football Player, turned College Football Coach. He is now a successful Entrepreneur who embodies the Warrior in a Garden ideology. I may be biased, but he is one of the toughest, most loving, and resilient men to walk this earth.

When dad was coaching Football as a Defensive Coordinator he used the Broad Axe to symbolize his defensive philosophy. He even had an axiom to outline it:

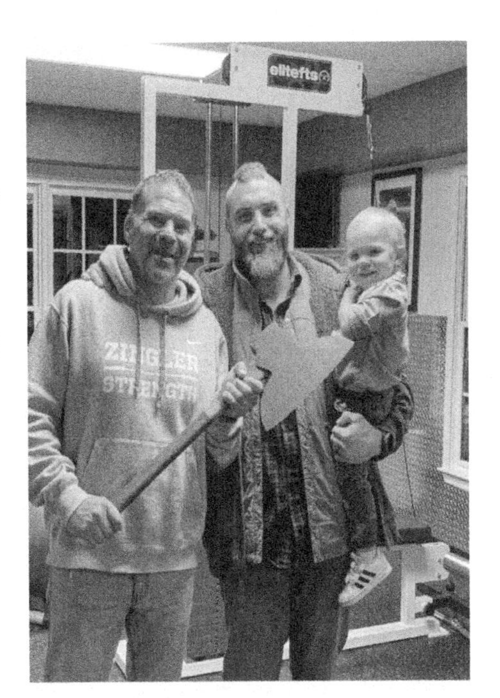

"There is nothing easy, nothing pretty about defense. It is a demanding taskmaster, a relentless taskmaster, and to be played well, it calls on a player to give up himself fully."

Sweat & Effort are its trademarks, and when forcefully applied, it is as blunt an instrument as an ancient Broad Axe."

This was the Creed of a Zingler Defense.

"Bring it from your shoes!" Dad would exclaim under full conviction before leading his guys onto the field.

I thought there was no better way to honor my father, who has given me everything, than to name this system after the instrument he held so dear. The instrument that is universally known to mean business.

The Broad Axe Training System is an efficient, frill-free approach to Strength & Conditioning. The system is designed to meet you where you are & is built on simple principles, fundamental exercises, and calculated, repeated efforts.

I do not know a lot, but I assure you this system will work, provided you do. Pop culture would lead you to believe otherwise, but hard work still works.

INTRODUCTION

"How can you tell which exercise is working unless you have the courage to cut down the number of exercises so you can figure out whether or not it actually works?" -Pavel Tsatsouline

I read a lot. I mean A LOT. I read quality literature damn near every day, but when I read that quote, in the form of a question, it hit me unusually hard. It spoke directly to me. Very rarely do you read something that has the ability to shift your entire mindset, but that simple quote I read several years ago changed my entire perspective on training.

Not to bore you to death with my life story, but at the time of this writing I've been training weekly for over 20 years and I have also been training a wide array of athletes, military personnel, and general populations since 2009 at the training facility I own, Zingler Strength & Conditioning.

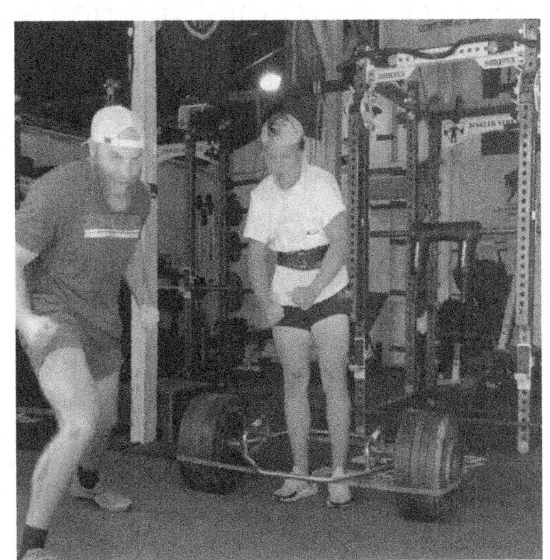

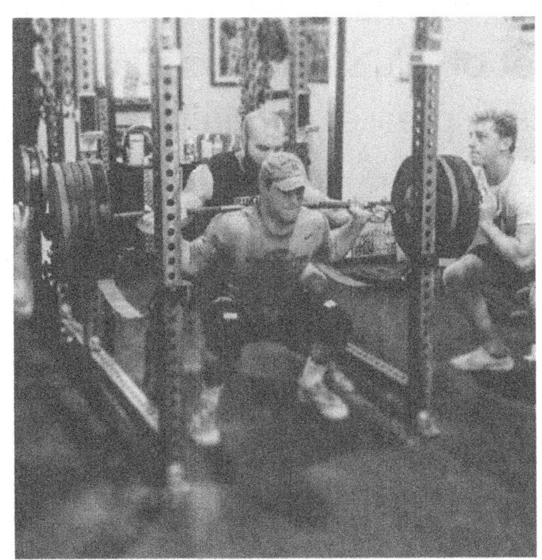

I have many thousands of hours training not only myself, but thousands of others in real life as well. I am not your stereotypical "buy my online program," guy.

When I began my training journey with my father back in the early 2000's it was initially to prepare me for sports.

I remember getting started with dad around 10 years old with the old school weight set many people had in that unfinished part of their basement. Hell, it might still be down there. I thought that was the coolest equipment in the world, until my life changed forever in the 8th grade.

One day before our 8th grade football season, dad took me down to the local fitness store and we bought a glorified training center. A squat rack, bench rack, smith machine, leg press/hack squat, lat pulldown machine, cable crossover, leg curl, leg extension, seated calf raise, and a dip station. We added our plates, barbells, and weight trees, and we had a home gym that would have rivaled anybody's back in the day. I named it "Metroflex Jr." That 434sqft. room would come to change my life forever.

Dad, who has always had a love for the iron game, trained me up using a lot of 'old school' training methods. We did a lot of high rep sets of bench presses, lat pulldowns, curls, squats, leg presses, hamstring curls and the like. We hammered out our sprints and stairs, too.

Like any teenager with testosterone coursing through his veins, I got strong. I mean damn strong, training this way.

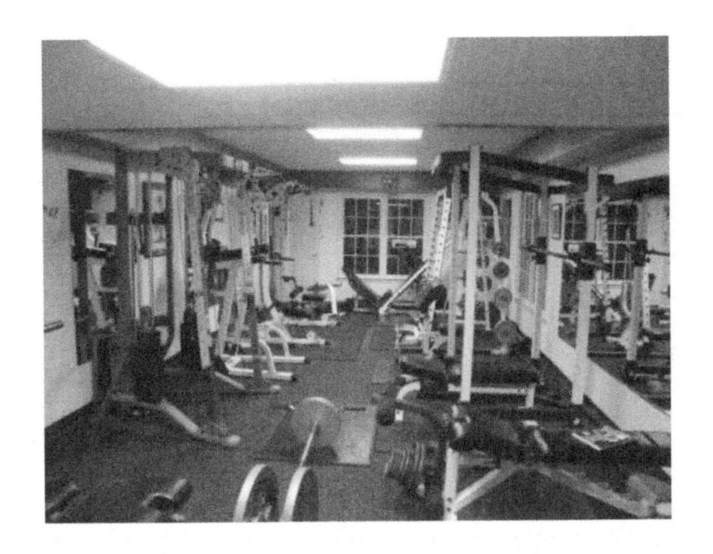

It was around 16 years old that I became obsessed with training.

Not like, "I really enjoy this training thing!", but "sorry I can't hang out after our football game on Friday night, I have to train legs."

After our football game, I'd crush a large pizza or two in the field house, come home, shower, throw on a pair of boxer briefs like an 80s bodybuilder and start my high-volume leg session in the basement around midnight.

At 16, I didn't understand why mom was so frustrated with me all the time, but it might have had something to do with blaring "let the bodies hit the floor" at max volume at 1am, before my heavy sets of squats.

Couldn't she just have understood I was only blaring 'Drowning Pool' for my top sets? She never did.

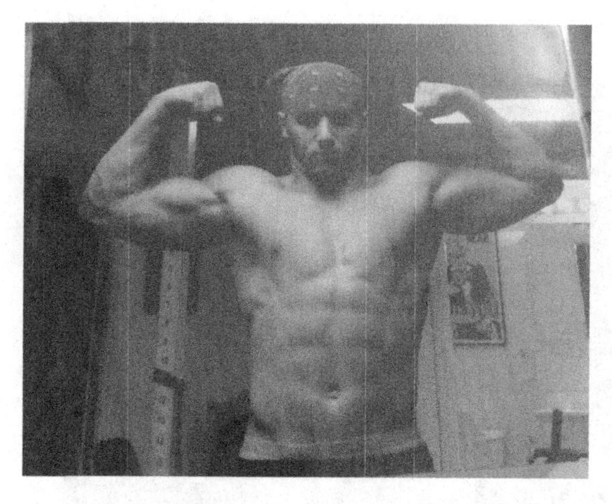

I can vividly remember pounding set, after set, after set, feeling like I could train all night. Those workouts would sometimes last 3 hours, and I loved every second of them.

As my training journey continued through HS, college, and beyond, I read a lot. I studied a lot. I trained A LOT. I've run many different programs myself over the years, but something I openly admit to doing with damn near all of them, is **ADDING** to them.

More is better, right?

Yep, as an immature trainee, I'd take Jim Wendler's 5/3/1 program or Joe DeFranco's Westside 4 Skinny Bastards program and follow them to a T, but then add 25%-50% volume to their programs, because after all "what the hell do these guys know, anyway?"

I was used to training 2+ hours a day, every day, and you're going to try to convince me that I can get a quality session in 30-45 minutes? No chance. I have watched Dorian Yates documentary 'Blood & Guts' too many times.

After years of adding volume to other genius programs that were written a certain way for a reason, I began to develop pain.

It started with little nagging elbow pain, then it was a little hip pain, but like any 'tough' guy, I'd brush it off and keep on, keepin' on.

And then it got serious.

I ripped a pec off the bone, developed distal clavicle osteolysis (bone chips in my shoulder), & suffered from hip pain that made me feel 70 years old at 25. I used to have to put my truck in park at redlights so I could quickly hop out and stretch my hips.

So what did I do? Stop? Of course not, I'd foam roll and do some mobility work to get some (VERY) temporary increased range of motion. Then I'd tape, brace, wrap, & strap, everything up as best I could to get through a session. I may or may not have added a shot of Jim Beam Whiskey to the mix to further numb the physical pain. HEALTH! Right?

It was around my mid 20's or so, while on the verge of mental and physical burnout that I decided there had to be a better way. I had spent so many years fighting the pain because I was under this illusion that this is just what you have to deal with to be big and strong.

I was on the brink of throwing in my training towel in my 'prime' because I'd literally & figuratively beat the shit out of myself. The thing (training) that I loved more than anything in the world was destroying me. And I wasn't even 30.

Several years ago, I stumbled on a book called Simple & Sinister by Pavel. It is a minimalist program of nothing more than Kettlebell Swings and Turkish Get Ups. Literally that's the entire program. I said to myself, I've always been the high volume, barbell or death junkie and had never really done a program like this, but I am going to sell out on this for 12 weeks. I was in so much mental and physical pain from my traditional training methods, I felt like I had no choice.

With my irrational fear of "losing all of my muscle mass" from not doing copious amounts of isolation work in tow, I embarked on the 12-week journey.

I finished the first day of 10x10 KB Swings & 10 Turkish Get Ups in about 25 minutes. I remember thinking, "What the hell? Is this it?"

I had committed to buying all the way into the program, so I reluctantly re-racked my kettlebells and hit the lights.

For the rest of that day I battled with myself to not go back in for more. I was stirred up like an addict waiting for the next day to come so I could get in another session.

Day 2 came and went and so did the many days after it.

After a few weeks of nothing but daily swings and get ups, something happened to my mind. I felt refreshed. I felt rejuvenated. Mentally and physically. I felt like I got a second wind.

There was no thought associated with training because the program was so simple, I'd go in, do my work, and get out. Sure I focused on each set and gave each one my best, but I was freed up from having to worry about 9 different exercises and 40+ sets.

It was one of the best programs I've ever run in my life. Not only did I not lose any muscle mass, I got stronger, I felt better, my body composition improved, and most importantly, my pain significantly diminished.

I said I'll be damned if there isn't something to this minimalist nonsense these Youtubers are talking about.

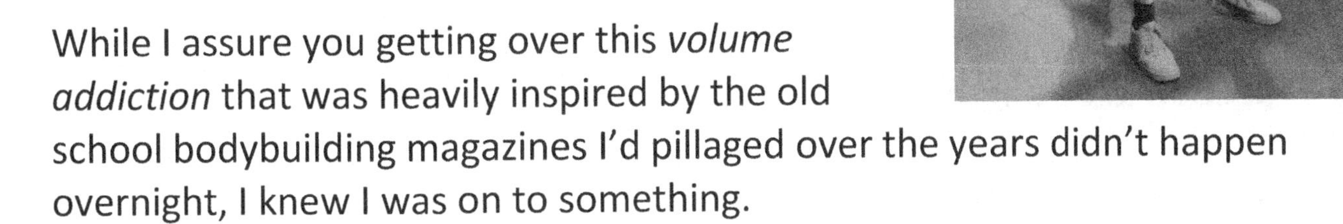

This put me in the front seat on the longevity bus and I've been searching for ways to adapt my traditional and preferred training styles ever since. I started asking myself questions like: "Is more really better? Or is it just more?" I've found out that only better is better.

While I assure you getting over this *volume addiction* that was heavily inspired by the old school bodybuilding magazines I'd pillaged over the years didn't happen overnight, I knew I was on to something.

I was and still am heavily influenced by guys like Louie Simmons, Jim Wendler, Joe DeFranco, Zach Even-Esh, Dan John, Pavel Tsatsouline, & Dave Tate. If I could go back, the only change I would make personally would have been to listen to their advice, not add more to it, falsely believing *more is better*.

If you're familiar with any of these legends of the iron game, you will quickly be able to pick up on how their influence on my life & training bleeds through this training system.

If you're unfamiliar with them, I would encourage you to look into their work as I am simply standing on their shoulders.

The goals of this system are to meet you where you're at on your strength and conditioning journey regardless if you're new to training or a high mileage trainee. To help you simply, safely, and effectively enhance your strength, conditioning, and body composition so that you can enjoy an increased overall preparedness for life.

This system is simple, but it isn't easy. More than anything it will ask for your discipline. Discipline to train consistently, yes, but also discipline to drown out the noise being shoved into your cranium by the "FitFluencers" on every social media app and street corner.

Buying into simple and mundane is real *hard* part.

This Book is laid out in 4 Sections:

Section 1: Strength

Section 2: Conditioning

Section 3: Diet, Supplements, Recovery

Section 4: Template Examples

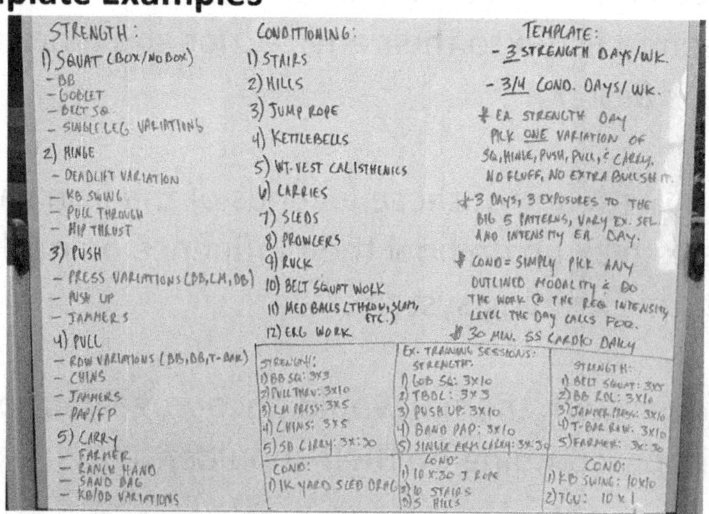

Section 1:

STRENGTH

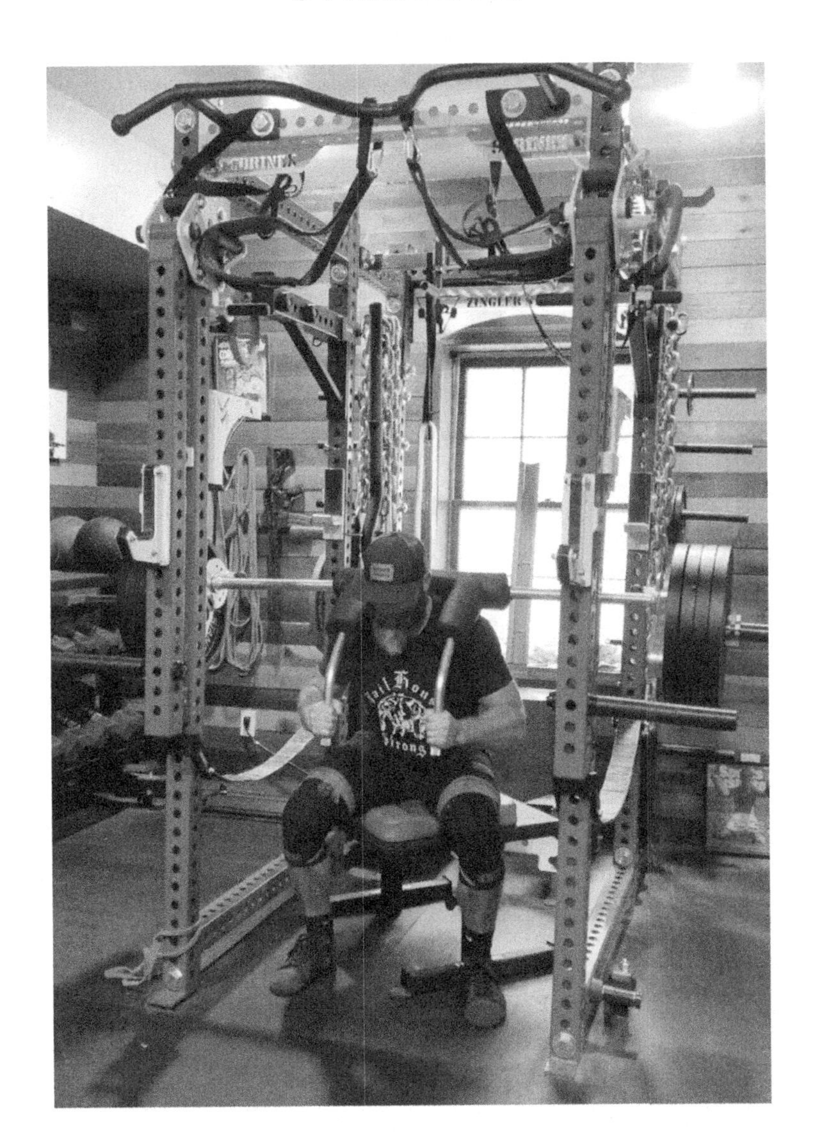

Chapter 1:

Nuts & Bolts

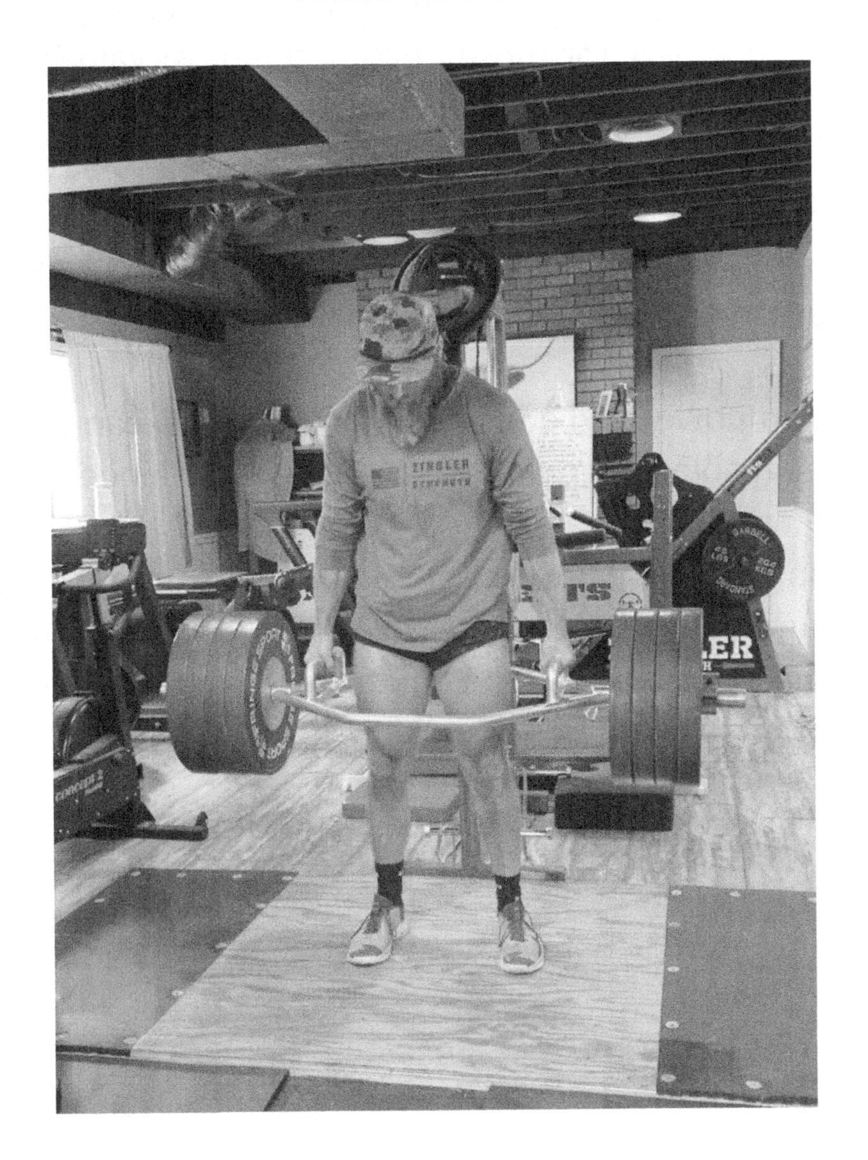

"Why are you calling it a system, Ray, can't you just give us the program?"

I assure you, in the coming pages, you'll *get the program* as well as several different variations of how to run it. The main reason I call it a system is because it is HIGHLY customizable and easy to adjust to meet the needs of any trainee.

While I know there are some people who just like to be given exercises, sets, and reps (it's there for those of you), the most valuable information I've ever received from a coach was the knowledge of how to develop a system.

Anybody can follow a spreadsheet with an 8-week program laid out and get results, but did you learn anything from it?

My goal is to empower and educate you so that you can become a more knowledgeable, independent, and creative trainee.

You're welcome to follow my templates, you can jump straight to the end if you want, but I would advise you to read this book in its entirety because by the end of it, you'll be equipped with the knowledge to design your own program.

Let's get started.

Getting Started: Squat, Hinge, Push, Pull, & Carry

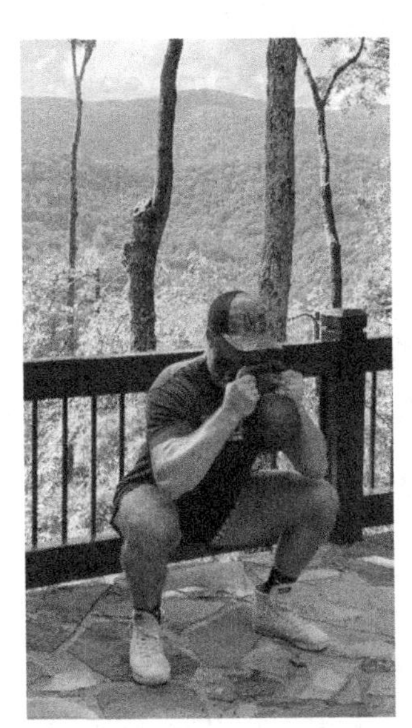

The Squat, Hinge, Push, Pull, & Carry are 5 fundamental patterns that you've likely performed if you've ever been in or around a weight room. Because you're reading this book, I would assume that you have. The hinge may be the most confusing one, but to clear it up, think hip hinge (Deadlift, RDL, KB Swing, etc.).

Of course I didn't invent these patterns. These patterns have been around forever and will continue to be around forever. This is the main reason I am using them for this system.

If anything in the training world has stood the test of this much time, I am willing to investigate it. I simply (and I'm not the first) decided to combine these 5 big patterns and perform them every training day.

The reason I chose these compound movements is because by themselves, they check a lot of boxes, when combined together, there aren't a whole lot of boxes, if any, they miss.

A lot of good can come from squatting weights, hinging weights, pushing weights, pulling weights, and carrying weights. These have long been staples for a reason.

I am not going to try to convince you of their value because in modern times this is common knowledge. Nor am I going to go through 100 different cues for each exercise. If you are unfamiliar or uncomfortable with any of the exercises, seek instruction from a qualified professional near you or, if you're looking for online coaching, feel free to reach out to yours truly.

While there will always be *that guy* who says, "you don't have to do squats," or "deadlifts are bad for you," do you really *have* to do anything? In my study of some of the greatest coaches and trainees in the world, the vast majority use these patterns.

Obviously if you have physical limitations or have been instructed by a medical professional to stay away from certain exercises, stay away from them. However, I've found that these patterns can be regressed and progressed to meet the needs of just about anyone.

Dan John, whom I recognized previously as having a tremendous influence on me is really big on the combination of these patterns as well. He has a program that is also one of my favorites called, 'Easy Strength'. Yep. It sounds like a *too good to be true* program, but it's not. I've done it. It's easy and it works.

He also has one of my favorite quotes regarding not only training, but life: "If it's important, do it every day."

While there have been many influences upon me, as well as many years of trial, injury, and error, searching for better ways, this system was born largely out of the two quotes shared in these initial pages.

I combined "How can you tell which exercise is working unless you have the courage to cut down the number of exercises so you can figure out whether or not it actually works?" + "If it's important, do it every day." This is how the Broad Axe Training System was born.

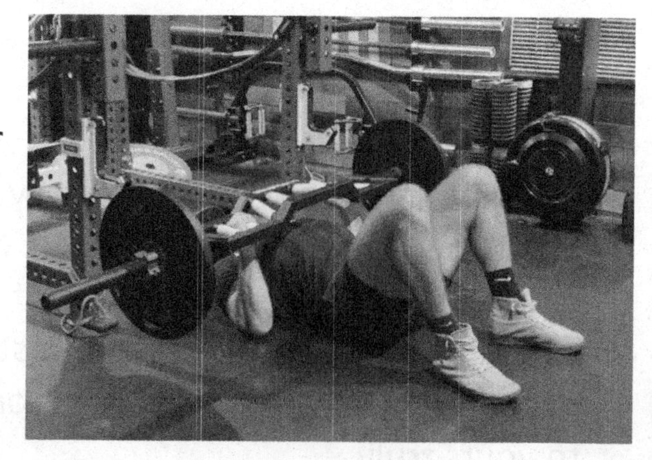

Strength Training

Strength is a relative term, right?

Strength can mean adding 10 pounds to a powerlifters squat max in a competition, but it can also mean improving your ability to manipulate your own bodyweight. Your body *is* weight, isn't it?

This system is designed to help you get stronger.

I believe every person on earth should be strength training in some capacity. From young kids to senior citizens, there is not a demographic on earth who cannot benefit from getting (relatively) stronger.

Goals, training styles, intensity, and frequency, can and should differ from person to person, but everyone should be getting themselves relatively stronger if they want to maximize their quality of life.

Strong people have a better quality of life than weak people. It's just the truth.

Despite coming from a background of extremely high-volume training (that I learned a lot of good & bad lessons from), this system is built on efficiency. You're not going to need to spend ridiculous amounts of time training to extract value from this system. This is a cut to the chase, get in & get out, program. While it doesn't require *hours* a day in the gym, it does ask for frequent, consistent training exposures.

Is this the best program for the ultra-competitive powerlifter or marathoner? Probably not, but I will tell you there is NO one size fits all perfect program. Anyone who tries to tell you there is, is lying. Every program has gaps, including this one, but I am certain it will serve a wide variety of people who are looking to get stronger and into better shape.

In the coming pages I will unbox the entire program for you. While there is a lot of information packed into these pages, recognize the system is wildly simple.

On your Strength Training days, you'll simply be picking 1 Squat Variation, 1 Hinge Variation, 1 Push Variation, 1 Pull Variation, and 1 Carry Variation, to perform on **every** Strength Training day.

I will explain how I recommend you run the system, but my ways are not the only ways.

This program can be performed by the greenest of beginners to the most advanced trainees on earth.

You can perform this program inside a world class, state of the art training facility, or with a medium sized rock in your backyard.

I've found the sweet spot for this program to be in the middle of the aforementioned extremes, using nothing more than common Strength Implements: Barbells, Dumbbells, Kettlebells, Bands, and etc.

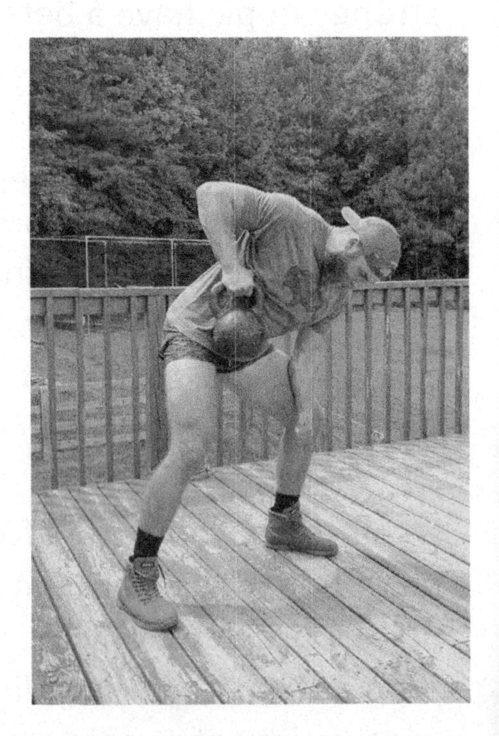

There are no secrets. There are no hidden exercises. There isn't *more* to it. You don't have to have 'x'. You just have to do the work. It is as straightforward as straightforward gets.

Chapter 2:

Training Frequency

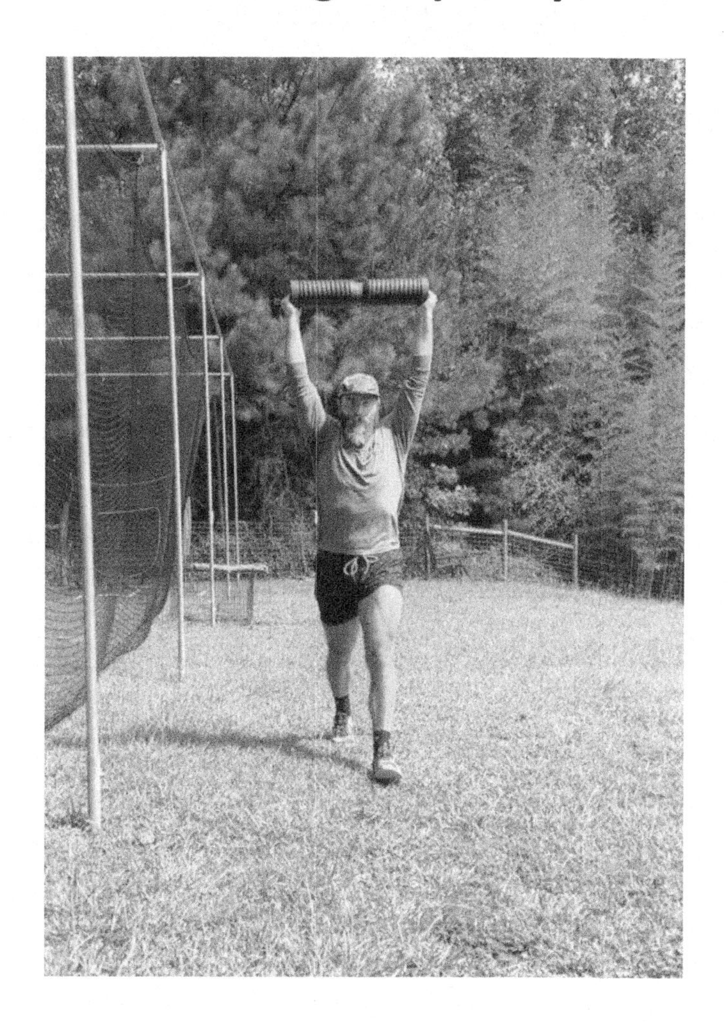

As I've gotten older, I have learned that consistency beats intensity. I've also learned the value of high frequency training. Personally speaking, though I believe many would agree, I prefer doing a little something every day over doing a whole lot of something a couple times per week.

The main outline of this system is written exactly how I prefer to program it for myself, 6 days per week of 25-45 minute sessions, with most sessions ranging in that 30-40 minute time range. Obviously if you choose a lower frequency template, that requires **both** Strength & Conditioning on the same day, your sessions may take a bit longer.

This said, I recognize that the majority of people who will be using this system may not have 6 days per week to commit to training, so I provide 2-5 day per week templates that will also work very well.

Because the sessions are relatively low in volume, I would encourage you to plan on training as many realistic days per week as possible as you will get the most benefit from consistent training exposures.

For this system, I would call 5-6 days/week ideal, 3-4 days great, & 2 days acceptable, but I recognize that everyone's situation is different and will always preach that some done often beats nothing done, ever.

*Note: This is a balanced program of 50% Strength exposures and 50% Conditioning exposures. Because we're in the Strength Section, the initial example templates will only have the **Strength** work listed. When you see "6-Day Template" this is referring to 3 Strength Days & 3 Conditioning Days. If you choose a '3-Day Template' you'd have 3 total training days, performing 3 Strength and 3 Conditioning sessions performed together, **6 Exposures** via **3 Total Sessions** per week.

Program Design

After you've decided on the realistic number of days per week you can/want to commit to training, it's time to start designing your program. (If you're caught between two choices, choose the lower one.)

For your program you're going to select:

-1 Squat Variation
-1 Hinge Variation
-1 Push Variation
-1 Pull Variation
-1 Carry Variation
For each of your strength training days.

*For your **Push/Pull** variations you can select **Horizontal** and/or **Vertical** variations. For Horizontal selections, think Bench Press and Rowing type exercises and for Vertical selections think Overhead Press and Lat Pulldown. You can program whichever variations best reflect your goals, however personally I prefer a blend of both horizontal and vertical variations.

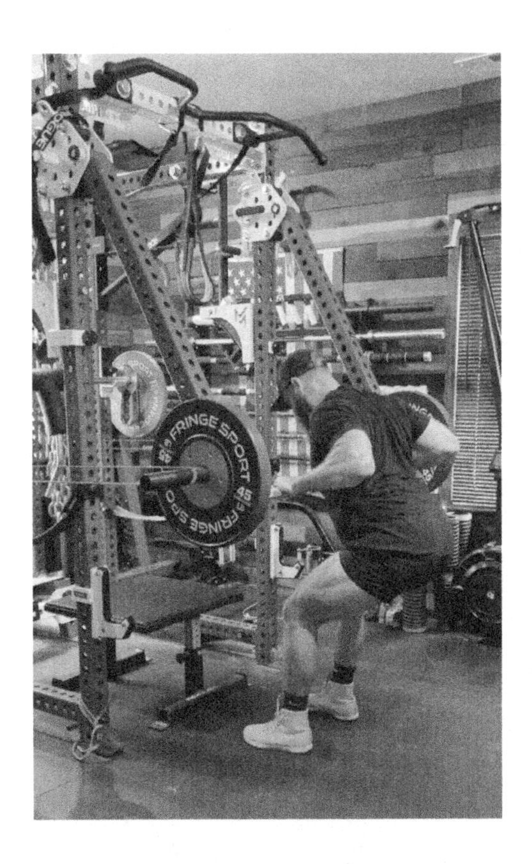

**All Templates, other than the 2 day/week template will have 3 Strength Days.

For the sake of explanation, I'm going to be referencing my **6-Day** Template, meaning 3 of my 6 days will be Strength Training days, however the concepts stay the same, despite the template you choose.

Day 1)

1. Squat Variation
2. Hinge Variation
3. Push Variation
4. Pull Variation
5. Carry Variation

Day 3)

1. Squat Variation
2. Hinge Variation
3. Push Variation
4. Pull Variation
5. Carry Variation

Day 5)

1. Squat Variation
2. Hinge Variation
3. Push Variation
4. Pull Variation
5. Carry Variation

3 Days. 5 Exercises per day. That's it.

*If you choose the 2 Day Template, it will look the exact same, with one less day.

There is no accessory work in addition (unless you want to add it in, though I don't advise it) to what you see. I recognize this style of training is likely different from what you are accustomed to, (traditional body part splits or traditional strength training prescription of main, assistance, & auxiliary lifts) but the idea of this program is to expose you to big, **full body**, meat and potato patterns, frequently and consistently.

Chapter 3:

Weights, Sets, & Reps

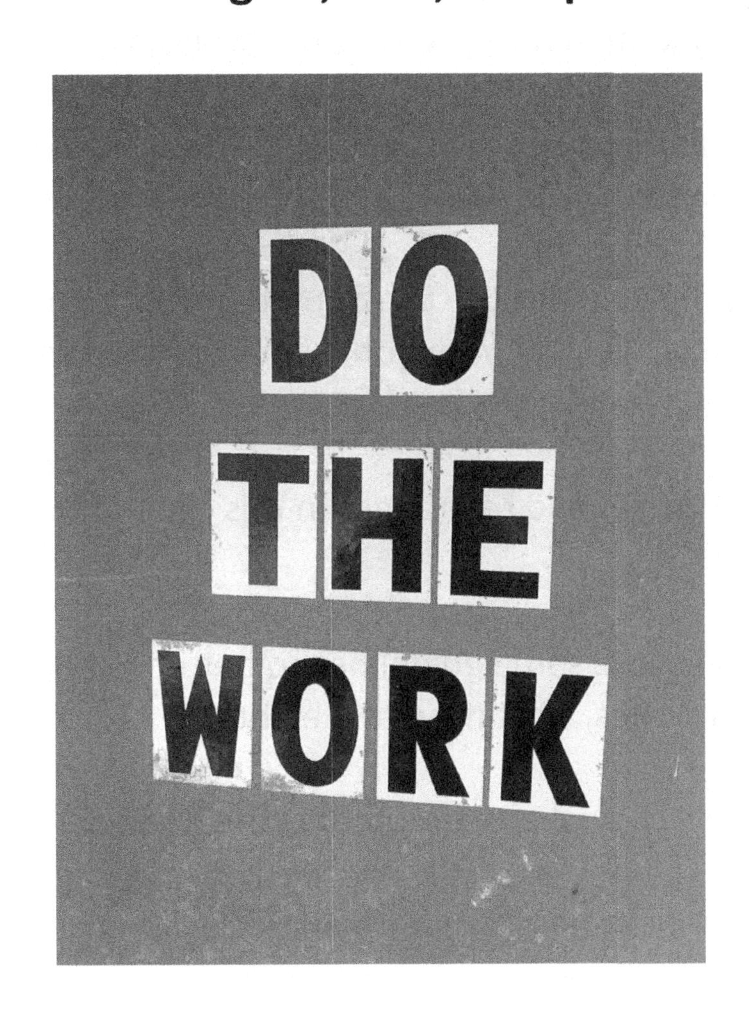

As I have shared a lot of training content on social media, the number one inquiry I get regarding the system is "well, what about weight, sets, and reps!?"

The weights, sets, and reps of this program can be highly volatile based on your preparedness levels, goals, access to equipment, time, etc.

Again, this is a system, not a "just do this" program.

I will say that regardless of the weights, sets, and reps you choose, the premise of the system is founded on the lifting of **submaximal weights**.

To clarify this simply means the use of moderate weights, not maximal, 95+ % of your max, weights. A major key to the program is WINNING every single set.

The recommended set and rep ranges in this program vary from **3-4 sets of 1-12 reps.**

I will unpack and share some guidelines to better help you choose weights, sets, and reps, starting with weights.

Before I get into it, I must share a bit of context as to how I got here.

The three most influential Strength Training Programs for me have and continue to be:

1) Jim Wendler's 5/3/1
2) Joe DeFranco's Westside 4 Skinny B*stards
3) Dan John's Easy Strength

The reason I highlight these incredible coaches again is because I must give credit where credit is due. Their influence on my training helped me to come up with the exercise selections, exercise variability, frequency, volume, intensities, and set and rep schemes.

While most are probably familiar with at least 1 and possibly all 3 of the programs, I am going to spell out my 2 recommendations of how to program weights, sets & reps for your Broad Axe System.

Easy Strength.

Dan John's Easy Strength program is fairly straightforward when it comes to choosing weights to use. Choose "Easy" weights.

Huh?

Yep, that's literally it. Based on the given set and rep schemes of the given exercise, choose weights that you know you can crush.

You're essentially training by *feel*.

For example, in the Broad Axe System, you'll see a set and rep scheme that might look like this: 3 sets of 5, 5, 5+.

What this means is you will perform **3 total sets**. 5 reps on your first set, 5 reps on your second set, and then on your 3rd and final set of 5+ reps (the **+** simply means **or more**) you have the option of simply hitting your 5 reps or performing As Many quality Reps As Possible (AMRAP).

It is best to start light and then progressively add each set, ensuring that on the last set you choose a weight you know you can perform for a **minimum** of all 5 reps. The idea is to **own** every set & never miss a rep.

Here's an Example:

Set 1: 225x5
Set 2: 255x5
Set 3: 275x5+ (If you have 7 quality reps in the tank at this weight and are feeling good, go get your 7, but do **not** get less than 5.)

If next week's set and rep scheme is 3 sets of 3, 3, 3+, again, you're performing 3 total sets and you'll want to choose a weight on your third set that you know you could perform for 4-6 reps. Own your set of 3, if you want to AMRAP your final set, go for it, just don't get anywhere near missing any of your prescribed reps.

This is my preferred way to program weights for this program because as you can see, it is very simple. You just simply and intelligently challenge yourself with weights you're confident you can handle. Just DON'T miss. I will refer to this method as the **By Feel Protocol.**

Despite preferring the By Feel Protocol, I know there are some of you out there who may not know how to feel out weights or you may desire to follow a percentage-based program.

I got you.

This is where Jim Wendler's **5/3/1 Protocol** comes into play.

If you're unfamiliar with Jim's work, I would encourage you to dig into it, however I will briefly explain the 5/3/1 Percentage Protocol over the next few chapters to help you prescribe specific weights to your program.

First, you need to find your current, not your "back in the day" maxes on whichever Main exercises you're going to be performing. This program will consist of Two *Types* of exercises, **Main** Exercises & **Aux** Exercises within your Squat, Hinge, Push, Pull, Carry, template.

More on the Main/Aux concepts later.

We need to know your Current Maxes so we can develop your **Training Maxes (TM)**. Training Maxes are a lesser percentage of your actual max. The idea of a Training Max is to give you an everyday number that you can hit despite feeling good, bad, indifferent, stressed, sick, or tired. You will be basing your programming off of your Training Maxes, not your true 1 Rep Maxes (1RM's).

For most, the Main exercises you will need Training Maxes for are the Barbell Squat, Deadlift, Bench Press and/or Overhead Press. You can find a Training Max for the Pull exercises within your program, but I've found this to be largely unnecessary as I recommend training the Pull as a *hybrid* Main/Auxiliary movement.

If you have current maxes, great. I am going to encourage you to take 80%-90% of your current max for each of your main lifts to create a Training Max.

Here is an example:

- Your Squat One Rep Max is – 315.

Now you are going to take 80%-90% of that number to get your Training Max. For example purposes, I am going to use 85% for the Training Max, though you can use any percentage within the range. **(Pro Tip: Aim Low)**.

To get your Training Max, simply multiply 315 x 85% (.85) = 270.

270 Pounds would be your Training Max for the Squat.

"I don't know my 1 rep maxes."

That's fine. You have 2 options.

Option 1:
Test yourself & find your 1RMs and then plug them into the Training Max calculator (1RM x .85 = TM)

Option 2 (Preferred Option): Estimate your 1RM.

To Estimate your 1RM pick a weight you KNOW you can handle for 3-5 reps. Perform a set of your **Testing Exercise**.

Now, let's use the Bench Press for example.

You put 225 on the bar and you get 4 reps. Awesome.

Now, use this formula to get to your estimated 1RM (this formula works fine for all exercise 1RM estimations):

Weight x Reps x .0333 + Weight =

Weight (225) x Reps (4) x .0333 + Weight (225) = ~255.

Your **estimated 1RM** for the Bench Press is **255 pounds**.

Now, simply multiply 255 x .85 (remember we're taking 80-90% of our estimated 1RM to get your TM) to get your Training Max of 215.

You would use **215 pounds** as your **Training Max** for the Bench Press.

Once you have your Training Maxes, you're ready to plug & play.

Chapter 4:

Mains & Auxiliarys

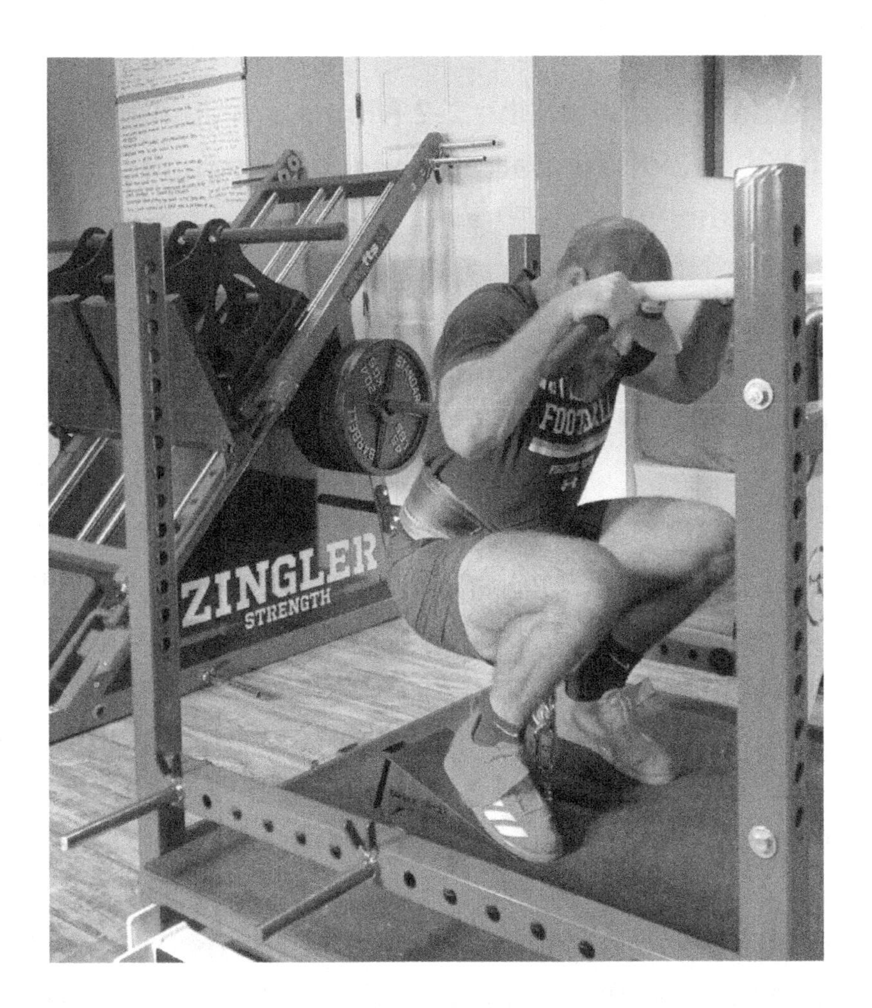

Before moving any further, I must explain the **Main** and **Aux** concepts. We've touched on the movement patterns, training frequency, weights, sets, & reps, now I'm going to touch on the Main and Aux concepts I briefly introduced in the previous chapter.

For each Strength Training Day, again, you will have programmed 1 Squat Variation, 1 Hinge Variation, 1 Push Variation, 1 Pull Variation, and 1 Carry Variation.

On each of the days there will be **1-2 Mains**, meaning of the 5 patterns being performed, 1-2 of the patterns will be the main focal point exercises for that day.

You will then have **1-3 Aux** patterns, meaning of the 5 patterns being performed, 1-3 of the patterns will be performed as Aux or Auxiliary exercises for that day.

All this means is that on each of the given training days, certain patterns on certain days are going to be programmed as Mains (i.e. Strength Focus – think 1-5+ rep ranges) and certain patterns on certain days are going to be programmed as Aux (i.e. Volume focus – think your 8-12 rep ranges). The only pattern that I program a bit differently is the Pull Variation. I still recommend having a Main Pull, but instead of the 1-5 rep range, I'll use a 5-8 rep range for most Main Pull variations.

Again, you will be performing the same 5 patterns, Squat, Hinge, Push, Pull, & Carry on all of your Strength Training days, the focus on each exercise will shift between Main & Aux depending on the day.

***All Carries in this program should be performed as Aux Finishers. Challenge yourself with the carries, but do not overdo them. I recommend a variety of different carries performed for time/distance.**

Depending on the Template you choose, I would encourage you to program your Main/Aux Selections as follows:

Template Options:

6 Day:
Day 1: Strength (Aux Focus on All Lifts)
Day 3: Strength (Squat/Push Main, Hinge/Pull Aux)
Day 5: Strength (Hinge/Pull Main, Squat/Push Aux)

5 Day:
Day 1: Strength (Squat Main, Hinge/Push/Pull Aux)
Day 4: Strength (Push/Pull Main, Squat/Hinge Aux)
Day 6: Strength (Hinge Main, Squat/Push/Pull Aux)

4 Day:
Day 1: Strength (Squat Main, Hinge/Push/Pull Aux)
Day 3: Strength (Push/Pull Main, Squat/Hinge Aux)
Day 4: Strength (Hinge Main, Squat/Push/Pull Aux)

3 Day:
Day 1: Strength (Squat Main, Hinge/Push/Pull Aux)
Day 3: Strength (Push Main/Pull Main, Squat/Hinge Aux)
Day 5: Strength (Hinge Main, Squat/Push/Pull Aux)

2 Day:
Day 2: Strength (Squat/Press Main, Hinge/Pull Aux)
Day 4: Strength (Hinge/Pull Main, Squat/Push Aux)

The Mains outlined above will be where you implement your By Feel or 5/3/1 Percentage Protocol. The exercises on those days will again be your **strength focused** lifts, while the Aux exercises will be focused on increased volume. Think **bodybuilding** if you will for the Aux work.

I still advise you to perform the patterns in order: Squat, Hinge, Push, Pull, Carry, regardless of which exercises are Main or Aux, however if you prefer to put the Mains first, that is fine, if you like to superset, superset. Just get the work in.

Training Cycles

The Broad Axe Training system is designed in 3-week cycles, which works perfectly with Jim Wendler's 5/3/1 Protocol. I wonder where I got that idea? Thanks Jim.

The first week of training, you'll see prescribed as 3 sets of 5, 5, 5+ reps for your Main Exercises.

If you're using the By Feel Protocol, simply progress weights each set depending on how you're feeling, ensuring that on your 3rd and final set you get at LEAST 5 reps. You're welcome to AMRAP your **LAST** set if you have more than 5 clean reps in the tank. Again, there are only two rules with the By Feel Protocol: 1) Work intelligently hard. 2) Don't miss. Easy enough.

If you prefer to use the 5/3/1 Percentage Protocol, I will explain how to program weights for your Mains.

You will take your Training Max for the given Main Exercise(s) and plug them in as follows:

*For example purposes, let's go back to the previous Squat example. We had a 1 Rep Max of 315, but a Training Max of 270. We will use our TM of 270 to help determine the weights we will use for our 3 working sets each week.

Week 1 Mains:

Set 1: 65% of your TM x5 reps (.65 x 270 = ~175). **175 x 5 reps.**

Set 2: 75% of your TM x5 reps (.75 x 270 = ~200). **200 x 5 reps.**

Set 3: 85% of your TM x5 reps (.85 x 270 = ~230). **230 x 5+ reps.**

*Remember, '+' simply means **'or more'**. Because the program is designed using submaximal weights, you should hit your numbers fairly easily. I strongly encourage you to AMRAP your **last set** when using the 5/3/1 Percentage Protocol to really push yourself on that last set. That said, the reps must be quality. Cease the set when you feel your technique is breaking down. Much like the By Feel Protocol, the only rule is that you **MUST**, at the very least, get your prescribed number of reps.

*If you miss reps, your Training Max is likely too high and you should lower it. If you're getting 10 or more reps on your **+** set, you can likely bump your TM a bit.

For the ensuing 2 weeks of the cycle your set & rep schemes for your Main lifts will look as follows:

Week 2 Mains:

3 sets of 3, 3, 3+ reps at 70%, 80%, & 90% of your TM.

Using again, our 270 Squat example TM, our sets & reps for week 2 would look like:

190x3, 215x3, 245x3+ (AMRAP on the last set).

As you can see the weights used are increasing from week 1 to week 2 & they will increase again from week 2 to week 3:

Week 3 Mains:

3 sets of 5, 3, 1+ reps at 75%, 85%, & 95% of your TM.

Using our 270 Squat example TM, our sets & reps for week 3 would look like:

200x5, 230x3, & 255x1+ (AMRAP on the last set).

*To rid any confusion, the Main exercises will always have **3 Total Working Sets.**

3 sets of 5, 3, 1+ =
Set 1: 5 reps
Set 2: 3 reps
Set 3: 1+ reps

It is **NOT** to be interpreted as 3 sets of 5 reps, 3 sets of 3 reps, & then 3 sets of 1+ reps (9 total sets).

To summarize, the 5/3/1 Percentage Protocol, if you choose to go this route:

- Find your 1RM or Estimated 1RM.
- Take **80%-90%** of that number (again, aim low) to find your Training Max.
- Use your Training Max to program your weights for your Main exercises.

Week 1: 3 sets of 5, 5, 5+ reps @ 65%, 75%, & 85% of your TM.

Week 2: 3 sets of 3, 3, 3+ reps @ 70%, 80%, & 90% of your TM.

Week 3: 3 sets of 5, 3, 1+ reps @ 75%, 85%, & 95% of your TM.

After each 3-Week cycle, I recommend implementing a **Deload** week. During a Deload week you will be using less volume and intensity for the purposes of giving yourself a recovery week. Deloading is optional, however for long term progress, I strongly encourage incorporating deloads.

At the start of your next training cycle (week 4 or 5) you will simply restart the percentage, set & rep scheme and add **10 pounds** to your Training Maxes (**not** your actual 1RM's) for your **lower body lifts** & **5 pounds** to your Training Maxes for your **upper body lifts**, provided you **didn't miss** any reps in your previous training cycle or **change** the Main exercise selection.

For the sake of our examples outlined above, your Squat Training Max would bump from 270 to 280 and your Bench Press Training Max would bump from 215 to 220. Then, you simply plug & play again.

Whether you choose the By Feel route or use the 5/3/1 Percentage Protocol, the program concepts stay the same. 1-5(+) reps for the Mains, 8-12 reps for the Auxs.

Each week, the reps on the Main exercises will decrease, so the weights should increase.

Each week, the reps on the Aux Exercises will increase. Use weights that are challenging, but be smart. The goal of the Aux exercises is to build quality volume (think hypertrophy training). You can record weights used for the Aux Exercises and try to progress them each week, however I prefer to train them By Feel.

*All Sets prescribed in the templates are working sets so take as many sets as you need to warm up. Because the program is submaximal by design you shouldn't need 5 warmup sets to get ready for your first working set.

Despite which route you choose for your program, you want to WIN, not win, but WIN every set.

Chapter 5:

Programming Notes

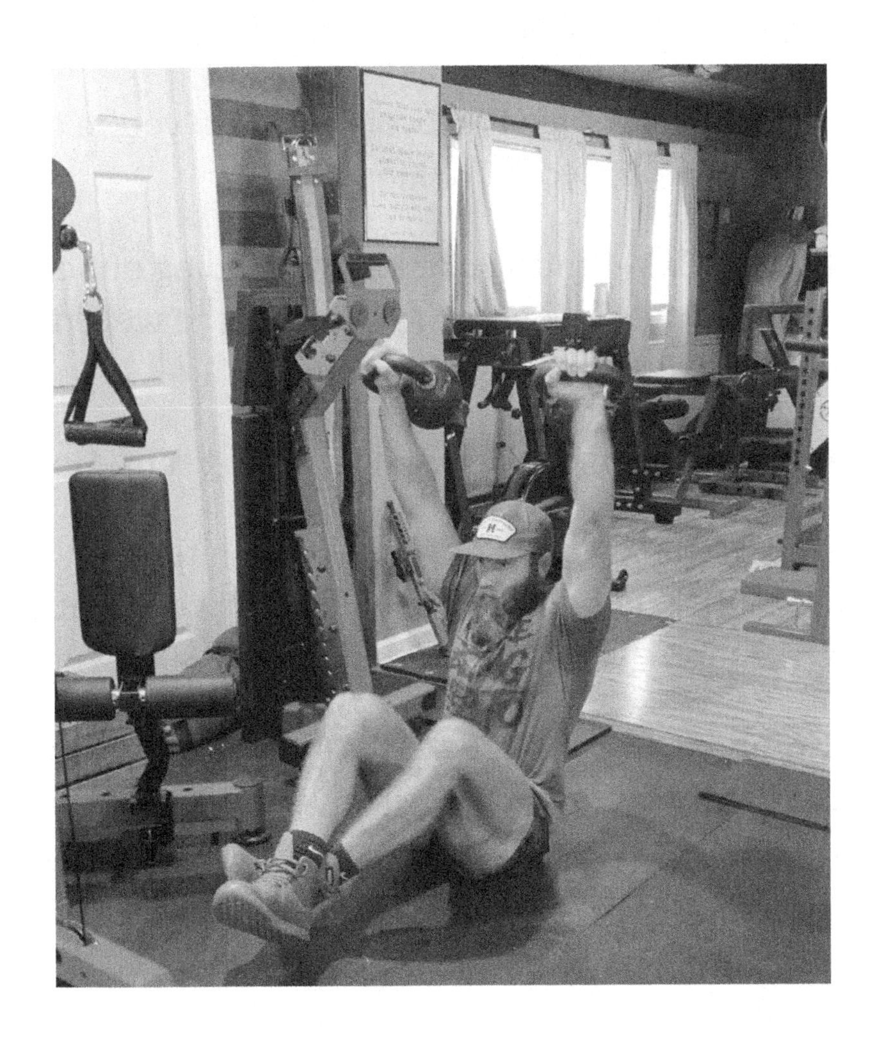

The idea of this program is to give more than it takes from you. The goal is to make steady, consistent progress, with submaximal weights so you're not consistently beating the shit out of yourself.

However, you do want to challenge yourself with quality effort each session.

If you choose the By Feel route and the rep scheme is 3x3+ and you pick a weight you could perform 14 times, it's too light.

If you go the 5/3/1 Percentage Protocol route and you're getting 16 reps on your 3+ set, adjust your Training Max.

If the rep scheme is 3x3+, and you're barely grinding out or missing the 3rd rep, regardless of the By Feel or 5/3/1 route, the weight is too heavy. Drop your ego &/or your Training Max.

I cannot overstress the importance of not missing reps. Don't miss.

You should be performing every single rep with intent. CRISP & STRONG lockouts, every time. A good rule of thumb is to know that at the very least you had 1-2 more (GOOD) reps in the tank.

While both methods DO work, the reason I prefer the By Feel route is because as the program moves along and your exercise selection varies (I recommend keeping all exercises the same for a **minimum** of 3 weeks) from cycle to cycle, your Training Maxes for exercise variations will shift.

For example, if you perform a 3-week cycle of Trap Bar Deadlift's and then you want to shift to a Straight Bar Deadlift for your next 3-week cycle, your TM from your Trap Bar will not carry over to the Straight Bar, meaning your numbers will be screwed up.

The same goes for your Back Squat TM & Safety Squat Bar TM. If you choose to implement different bars, variables, etc. from cycle to cycle, you must account for these changes as they will definitely impact your Training Maxes, which will ultimately impact your program.

If you are going to use the 5/3/1 Percentage Protocol I would encourage you to use LESS variability when it comes to exercise selection, especially on the Main exercises.

If you want to add variability, set your training maxes lower (65%-85%) so that the transition from bar to bar still allows you to WIN your sets and reps. There will be a bit of a learning curve here.

Unless you know your true 1RM (so you can get an accurate TM) for the different bars/variations you'll be using, the lesser variability option is a better choice for more consistent progress. Especially for beginners.

The reason the By Feel option works better here in my opinion is because despite changing from Straight Bar to Cambered Bar, to Safety Squat Bar, (if you choose to) from cycle to cycle, you can "feel out" each set.

If the rep scheme is 3x5+, start light on your first set, bump a touch on your second set, and then based on how your first 2 sets went, pick a weight for your 3rd set that you KNOW you can handle for 7-8 reps and hammer out your 5 reps, or, if you're feeling wild, as many quality reps as possible on that last + set.

Finally, & I know I am beating a dead horse here, whichever route you choose, the most important concept is that you do **NOT** miss. WIN every set.

Choosing Mains and Auxs

As you're designing your program or using the templates provided in the final section, you'll want to be strategic about what exercises you choose for your Main and Aux Selections.

I don't really care which exercises you choose as you can essentially set it up however you want, but something to consider:

When choosing exercises I encourage you to think "**Main = Big** and **Aux = Smaller**".

What I mean by this, is your Barbell Squat Variations, Barbell Deadlift Variations, Barbell Press Variations, and Barbell Row Variations are going to be better Main selections and your Goblet Squats, KB Swings, Push Ups, & Face Pulls are going to better Aux Selections.

Push Ups, while a phenomenal exercise, aren't going to be the best choice as a Main Push for most, because 3 sets of 3 push-ups isn't going to be enough volume, but Push Ups as an Aux Exercise? 4 sets of 12? This is a much better prescription for most.

Again, this is totally up to you as the individual, so plug and play how you best see fit, I just feel some variations serve better as Mains and some serve better as Auxs.

Another thing you must consider is your preparedness level. If you have not been doing a lot of Barbell work recently, programming a bunch of Barbell Squats & Barbell RDL's multiple days per week will leave you feeling very sore.

You'll notice in my example templates I only have **1** Barbell Squat Variation each week placed on my Main Squat Day. The other two variations are Belt Squats & Goblet Squats (No spinal loading). Program *easier* variations at first & then build yourself up. If you have a lot of experience with the Barbell, feel free to program it as much as you want.

Below are examples of programming one **Big** Compound for each of the training days per week.

As you progress and adapt to the training, you can add in more Barbell work. Be honest with where you're at and set yourself up to win the long game. The smaller variations are extremely valuable. They are highly recoverable and will assist your strength development and enhance your work capacity. Remember, the name of this game is highly frequent, lower volume exposures. Don't beat yourself up.

3 Squat Days/wk: Belt Squat, **Barbell Squat**, Goblet Squat
3 Hinge Days/wk: DB RDL, **BB Deadlift**, KB Swing
3 Push Days/wk: DB OH Press, **BB Bench Press**, Push Ups
3 Pull Days/wk: Lat Pulldown, **Bent Over Row**, DB Row

*For the Carry, I will typically program 1 *Heavy* Carry & two *Smaller* Carries:

3 Carry Days/wk: KB Single Arm, **Heavy Sandbag**, 'Bottoms Up' KB

Here are some example templates of what each Strength Day would look like with actual exercises programmed based on the outline from above.

Remember your Aux Exercises are going to be your 3-4 sets of 8-12 and your Main Exercises are going to be your 3 sets of 1-5+, with the exception of Pull Mains, I typically encourage waving the reps something like 8-5, over 3 weeks. If you prefer to program them like the rest of the Main's that is fine, too.

6 Day Template (3 Strength Days)

Strength Day 1

1. Belt Squat (Aux)
2. DB RDL (Aux)
3. Incline Dumbbell Press (Aux)
4. Dumbbell Row (Aux)
5. Farmer Carry (Medium Intensity)

Strength Day 2

1. Barbell Back Squat (Main)
2. KB Swing (Aux)
3. Bench Press (Main)
4. Band Face Pull (Aux)
5. Suitcase Carry (Medium Intensity)

Strength Day 3

1. Goblet Squat (Aux)
2. Conventional Deadlift (Main)
3. Incline DB Press (Aux)
4. Bent Over Row (Main)
5. KB Goblet Carry (Medium Intensity)

With the 6-Day Template, Day 1's exercises will all be Aux based, 3-4 sets of 8-12 reps per exercise.

The idea here is to start the week off nice and easy. The goal is to *grease the groove* and prepare for the training week ahead. Going for broke on the first day of the week usually isn't the best idea as this will likely inhibit performance as the training week progresses.

Get in. Punch the clock with modest weights. Get out.

Day's 3 & 5 will follow the Main/Aux Protocol.

3, 4 & 5 Day Template (3 Strength Days)

Strength Day 1

1. Barbell Back Squat (Main)
2. DB RDL (Aux)
3. Incline Dumbbell Press (Aux)
4. Dumbbell Row (Aux)
5. Farmer Carry (Medium Intensity)

Strength Day 2

1. Belt Squat (Aux)
2. KB Swing (Aux)
3. Bench Press (Main)
4. Bent Over Row (Main)
5. Suitcase Carry (Medium Intensity)

Strength Day 3

1. Goblet Squat (Aux)
2. Conventional Deadlift (Main)
3. Incline DB Press (Aux)
4. Band Face Pull (Aux)
5. KB Goblet Carry (Medium Intensity)

The 3, 4, & 5 Day Templates have some slight variation to them as the first training day of the week will ask for 1 Main (Squat), and the rest of the lifts will be Aux.

The second Strength Day of the week calls for Push/Pull Mains & Squat/Hinge Aux.

The Last day of the week calls for a Hinge Main, & Squat, Push, Pull Aux.

The reason I set it up this way is because based on the template you choose, there will be some conditioning baked into certain days on any template **less** than 6 days.

It works out to look like:

- A Squat Main Day.
- A Push/Pull Main Day.
- A Hinge Main Day.

You can modify it however you want; this is just what I have personally found to work best on the lower frequency template options.

2 Day Template (2 Strength Days)

Strength Day 1

1. Barbell Back Squat (Main)
2. KB Swing (Aux)
3. Bench Press (Main)
4. Band Face Pull (Aux)
5. Suitcase Carry (Medium Intensity)

Strength Day 2

1. Goblet Squat (Aux)
2. Conventional Deadlift (Main)
3. Incline DB Press (Aux)
4. Bent Over Row (Main)
5. KB Goblet Carry (Medium Intensity)

This template is identical to the 6-day Template (3 Strength Days), outside of obviously missing an additional training day.

I put the Squat/Press together as Mains as well as the Hinge/Pull. If you prefer to program Squat/Hinge Main on Day 1, & Push/Pull Main on Day 2, go right ahead. I just like separating the big Lower Body Mains when possible.

Later in the example template you will see exactly how I lay out each of the 3-week cycles (4 weeks if including the Deload) but for further clarification here is an example of how each cycle looks should you choose the 3-, 4-, or 5-Day Template:

Day 1

1. Barbell Back Squat: W1: 3x5+, W2: 3x3+, W3: 3x5,3,1+, W4: D
2. DB RDL: W1 3x10, W2: 4x10, W3: 4x12, W4: D
3. Incline Dumbbell Press: W1: 3x10, W2: 4x10, W3: 4x12, W4: D
4. Dumbbell Row: W1: 3x10, W2: 4x10, W3: 4x12, W4: D
5. Farmer Carry: W1: 3x:30, W2: 3x:40, W3: 3x:45, W4: D

Day 2

1. Belt Squat: W1: 3x10, W2: 4x10, W3: 4x12, W4: D
2. KB Swing: W1 3x10, W2: 4x10, W3: 4x12, W4: D
3. Bench Press: W1: 3x5+, W2: 3x3+, W3: 3x5,3,1+, W4: D
4. Bent Over Row: W1: 3x8+, W2: 3x5+, W3: 3x5+, W4: D
5. Suitcase Carry: W1: 3x:30, W2: 3x:40, W3: 3x:45, W4: D

Day 3

1. Goblet Squat: W1: 3x10, W2: 4x10, W3: 4x12, W4: D
2. Conventional Deadlift: W1: 3x5+, W2: 3x3+, W3: 3x5,3,1+, W4: D
3. Incline DB Press: W1: 3x10, W2: 4x10, W3: 4x12, W4: D
4. Band Face Pull: W1: 3x10, W2: 4x10, W3: 4x12, W4: D
5. KB Goblet Carry: W1: 3x:30, W2: 3x:40, W3: 3x:45, W4: D

Below are example exercises for the Squat, Hinge, Push, Pull, & Carry patterns you can choose from. This is not a comprehensive list, but I believe this list will give you plenty of choices to choose from. I will also acknowledge them with an "M" or an "A" to signify my personal preference of the exercises being better suited as Main Exercises or Auxiliary Exercise selections, but these concepts may shift for you depending on how you choose to run your program.

Squat:

1. Barbell Back Squat (M)
2. Barbell Front Squat (M)
3. Barbell Box Squat (all box heights) (M)
4. Specialty Bar Squats (SSB, Spider, Camber, etc.) (M)
5. Belt Squat (M or A)
6. Hack Squat (A)
7. Landmine Squat (M or A)
8. Machine Squats (A)
9. Bodyweight Squat (A)
10. Sissy Squat (A)
11. Single Leg Squat (A)
12. DB Squat (A)
13. KB Squat (A)
14. Sandbag/Odd Object Squat (M or A)
15. Pause Squat (M or A)
16. Speed Squat (M)
17. Tempo Squat (M or A)
18. Accommodating Resistance/Assistance Squat (M or A)

*If you can't squat, choose exercises that mimic the squat's benefits. Do what you can.

Hinge:

1. Conventional Deadlift (M)
2. Trap Bar Deadlift (M)
3. Sumo Deadlift (M)
4. KB Deadlift (A)
5. Sandbag Deadlift (M or A)
6. Romanian Deadlift (M or A)
7. Landmine Deadlift (A)
8. Good Mornings (M or A)
9. Kettlebell Swings (A)
10. Kettlebell Hinge (A)
11. Cable Machine Hinge (A)
12. Hinge Based Machines (M or A)
13. Glute Bridges (A)
14. Hip Thrusts (M or A)
15. Deficit Deadlift (M)
16. Block Deadlift (M)
17. Rack Pull (M)
18. Pause Deadlift (M)
19. Speed Deadlift (M or A)
20. Accommodating Resistance/Assistance Hinges (M or A))

Push:

1. Push Up Variations (A)
2. Barbell Bench Press (M)
3. Barbell Incline Bench Press (M)
4. Barbell Floor Press (M)
5. DB Bench Press (A)
6. DB Incline Bench Press (A)
7. DB Floor Press (A)
8. Barbell Overhead Press (M)
9. DB Overhead Press (A)
10. Arnold Press (A)
11. Push/Press Machines (M or A)
12. Landmine Press (M or A)
13. Jammer Press (A)
14. Dips (A)
15. Board Press (M or A)
16. Pause Press (M or A)
17. Speed Press (M or A)
18. Spoon Press (A)
19. JM Press (M or A)
20. Accommodating Resistance/Assistance Presses (M or A)

Pull:

1. Chin Up (M or A)
2. Pull Up (M or A)
3. Barbell Bent Over Row (M)
4. Inverted Grip Barbell Row (M)
5. Chest Supported Row (A)
6. Seal Row (M or A)
7. Row Machines (A)
8. Pendlay Row (M or A)
9. T-Bar Row (M or A)
10. Landmine Row (M or A)
11. DB Row (A)
12. Kroc Row (A)
13. Gorilla Row (A)
14. Lat Pulldown (A)
15. Low Row
16. Straight Arm Pulldown (A)
17. DB Pullover (A)
18. Bodyweight Row (Rings/Trx/etc.) (A)
19. Face Pull (A)
20. Pull-a-Part (A)

Carry:

1. Farmers Carry
2. Ranch Hand Carry
3. Kettlebell Carry
4. Dumbbell Carry
5. Barbell Carry
6. Trap Bar Carry
7. Suitcase Carry
8. Sandbag Carry
9. Rock Carry
10. Odd Object Carry

Chapter 6:

Strength Wrap Up

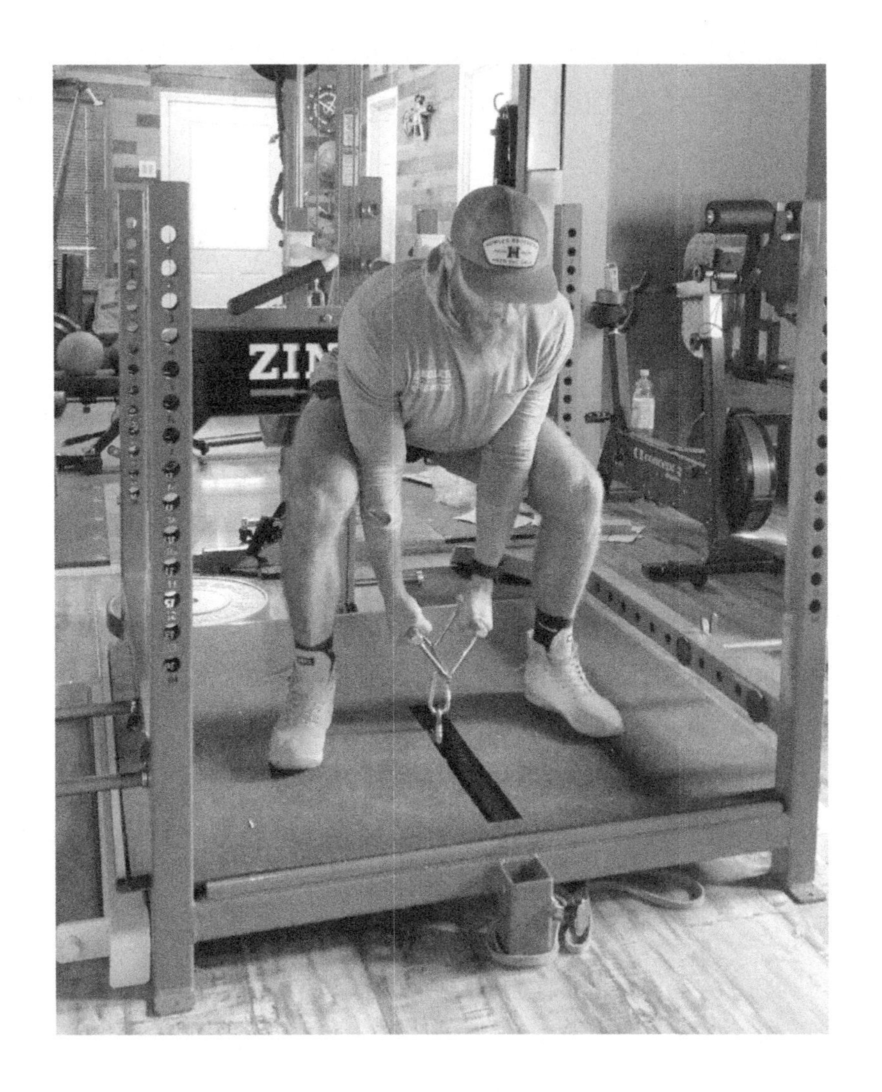

I know there is a lot of information in this strength section. My goal was to be as clear, repetitive, and simple as possible. If you have trouble understanding any of the information presented, it will be made clear in the example training templates provided at the end.

You'll also notice I didn't mention anything about warming up/mobility. The reason is because I have found warmups to be highly personal.

Personally speaking, I walk on the treadmill for 10 minutes, and then perform 2-3 rounds of goblet squats, leg curls, 45-degree back raises, & face pulls.

This may be great for you. You may need more; you may need less. Do what works for you.

If you're adamant about following a specific mobility routine, I'd point you to Joe DeFranco's Limber 11, it can be found online and is a phenomenal pre-training routine.

In Summary this program is nothing more than a Squat, Hinge, Push, Pull, and Carry every Strength Training Day, with varying set & rep schemes based on the given day (Mains & Auxs).

- Mains = 3 sets of 1 rep to 5+ reps. (*Pull pattern I will work up to sets as high as 8 on Main Day's).

- Auxs = 3-4 sets of 8-12 reps.

The program works in 3-week cycles (4 weeks including the Deload week).

Week 1: Mains are 3 sets of 5, 5, 5+, & Auxs are 3 sets of 10.

Week 2: Mains are 3 sets of 3, 3, 3+, & Auxs are 4 sets of 10.

Week 3: Mains are 3 sets of 5, 3, 1+, & Auxs are 4 sets of 12.

Week 4: Deload week. You can perform the same exercises as weeks 1-3 with reduced volume & intensity.

Week 5: Restart a new cycle (3-week wave). You're welcome to adjust some or all of the exercises from the previous training cycle. Depending on your training experience, I would keep the variability low if you're a beginner, and higher if you've got several training years under your belt.

If you're using the 5/3/1 Percentage Protocol and you do not change your Mains, increase your Upper Body TM's 5 pounds & Lower Body TM's 10 Pounds, then simply plug and play again. If you do adjust your Main exercise selection after each cycle, you must account for the variability in your Training Maxes.

Regardless of the By Feel or 5/3/1 Protocol I would encourage you to keep a training journal to track your progress. Record the weights used and rep maxes on your AMRAP sets. You don't have to max out every other week to see progress. If you hit 225 x 5 on Week 1 and then you hit it for 8 reps on Week 9, you're getting stronger. Call me Einstein.

I must remind you this is only a template. These are nothing more than guidelines and recommendations. You will need to make informed, honest decisions based on where you're at in **your** strength journey.

If I've encouraged 4 sets of 10 and you program 4 sets of 8 is it going to bastardize the program? Not at all. Maybe you're just starting out and can only do 2 sets of 10? Maybe your work capacity is on the higher end and you can benefit from 5 sets?

Use your judgment and stick to the Main/Aux Principles.

Performing these 5 patterns 2-3x a week over a consistent period of time is going to yield results.

I don't care if you only have a single Barbell and a couple plates or a single 53-pound Kettlebell. (I'll include a minimalist template in the template section.)

Run the damn program. I've done it with minimal equipment like this and it's worked tremendously.

Sure, you might have to adjust a few variables (sets, rep ranges, tempos, iso holds, etc.) if you have minimal equipment, but the program is designed to work, as long as you do.

KB Goblet Squat – 4x10
KB Swing – 4x10
KB Overhead Press – 4x10
KB Row – 4x10
KB Carry – 3x:45

Run a program like that 3 days a week, every week, for 16 weeks, adding reps, pauses and/or adjusting tempos each week. Sure it may not be the most exciting training prescription, but watch what happens.

I've run the program a variety of ways, using Training Maxes as low as 50-60 percent & still made tremendous progress.

For example, I hadn't squatted over 400 pounds in 5+ years because of all the wear and tear I developed in my joints over the years of beating the shit out of myself. Squatting remotely heavy just hurt too bad for the longest time, it was hell.

In a recent cycle of my Broad Axe Training, I never touched above 325 for any amount of reps on any Squat variation, but when I would work up to 325 I would smoke it with intent. (Remember it's important to own every set.)

Towards the end of one of my cycles I was feeling pretty good and said what the hell, I'll put 365 on the bar – smoked it for 5. Then I went ahead and stacked 4 plates on the SSB, again, not having felt this kind of weight in half a decade. I took 415 down to a box and it about scared me with how quickly it moved back up. I racked it after 3 blazing fast reps, but know I probably had 10+ in me.

The point of this story is not to brag about my squat strength. I have colleagues who can squat a grand +, what the hell is 400 pounds? The point of the story is that the consistent, mundane, repetition of crushing submaximal weights over long periods of time added up for me and it will for you too.

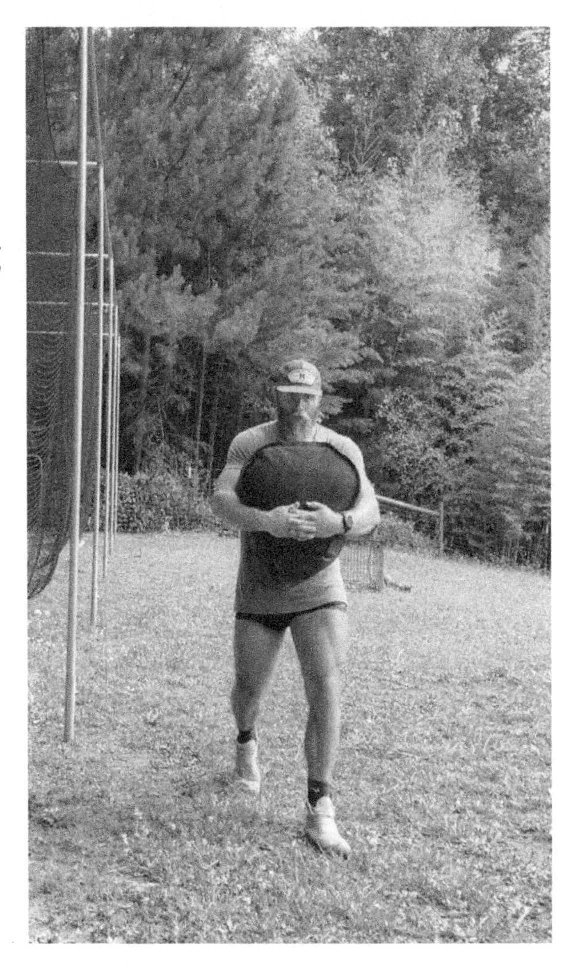

Punch the clock. Check the box. Leave some (plenty) in the tank. Then, simply repeat.

I promise that's all there is to it.

In the next section I will go over the Conditioning Principles of the Program.

SECTION 2: Conditioning

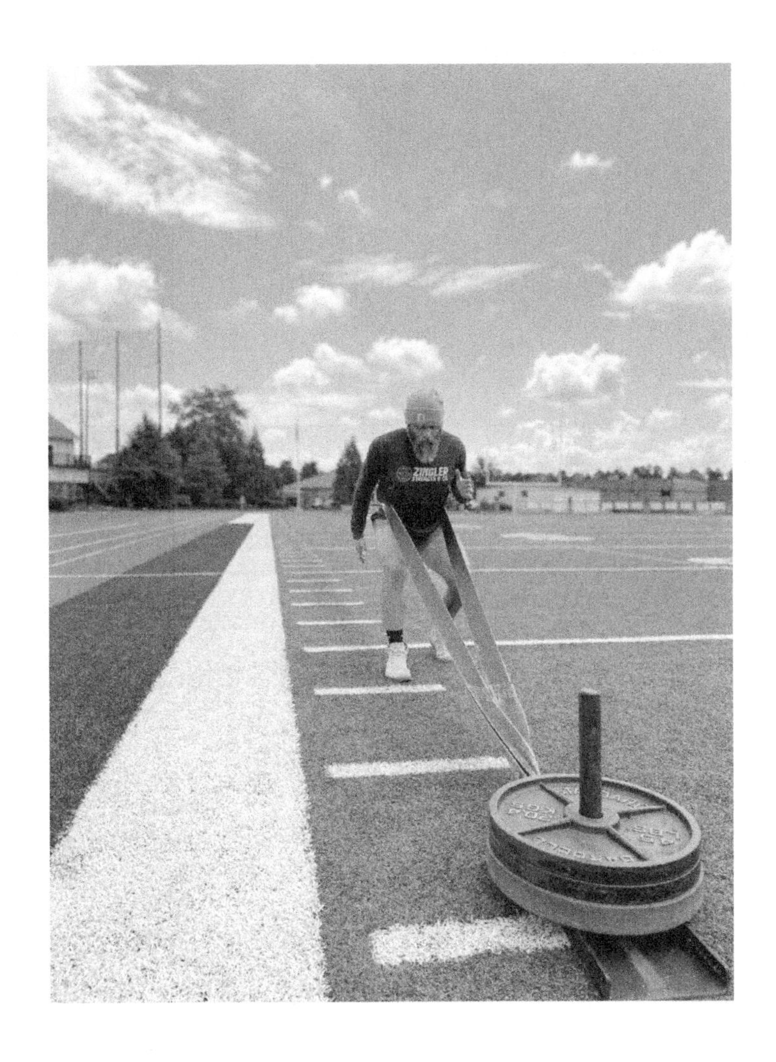

Chapter 7:

It's called Strength AND Conditioning

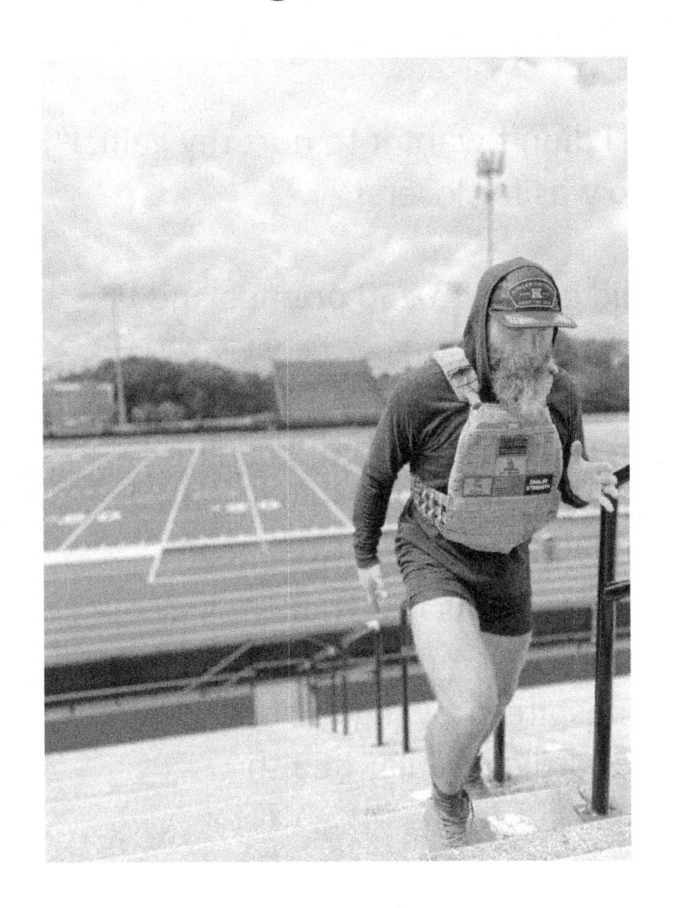

When I decided to hang up my cleats after high school and jump into a career in Strength & Conditioning, my own personal training looked more like STRENGTH & conditioning than it did Strength & Conditioning.

Okay, I'll just be honest, from 18-25, I did next to nothing for conditioning outside of intermittently pushing a Prowler a few times a year and then complaining about how awful it was.

This was because "I didn't want it to hurt my gainz!", "I wanted to be huge!" and "Cardio was for losers!"

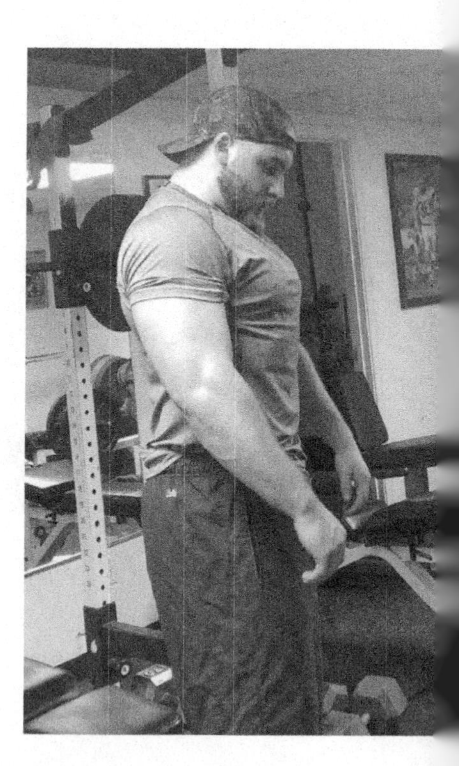

Let me tell you, I did get up to 250 pounds and I was strong as an ox, but it came at a cost.

I was only strong in the weight room, I couldn't make it up the stairs without losing my breath, I felt like hell, and my bloodwork in my mid 20s, even as a drug free lifter, was less than stellar. "I'll make a change later." I'd regularly catch myself saying this despite knowing I needed to start improving my cardiovascular health immediately.

In my mid 20's, I heard Mark Bell, a prominent figure in the industry, talking about 10-minute walks to improve his conditioning and mental health, so one day I said what the hell and started walking.

Then I woke up the next day and started walking again, and before too long, I found my conditioning calling. Walking. I could justify walking, because surely walking wasn't going to kill my gainz, was it?

Chalk, blood, and guts in the weight room in the mornings, & leisure walker in the evenings.

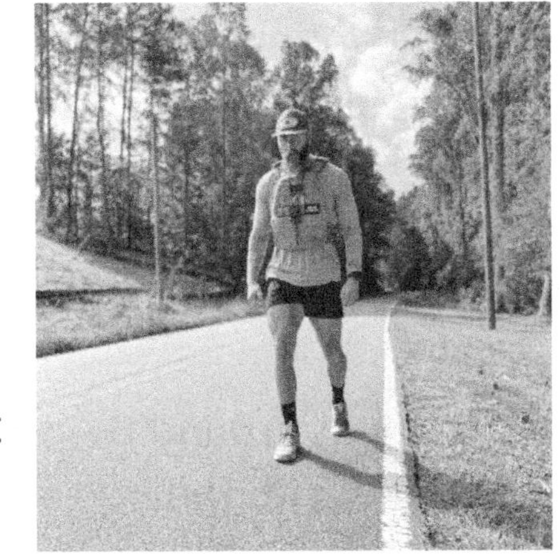

Walking was and still is the most underrated form of cardio of all time.

I remember being all excited to tell my buddies about my "brand new" discovery and how I thought it would help them too. They thought it was crazy that I was out going for walks.

To this day, I get calls from those same 'meathead buddies' who are slowly picking up on the value of walking.

While walking certainly isn't going to solve all the world's problems, I slowly started to watch it improve my work capacity and **General Physical Preparedness (GPP)** levels.

GPP is nothing more than your general state of physical preparedness. When I refer to GPP, I'm simply referring to your *state* of readiness for sport, life, etc. When we increase our preparedness levels through general training, we increase our ability to handle stress. Training, much like a workplace conflict, is stress.

I noticed in my strength training sessions, I moved faster, I didn't need to rest as long in between sets and I was just generally starting to feel better overall.

I began to think, what if I started doing more of this conditioning stuff? And then I'd quickly shut the idea down because I'd remind myself "I'm a lifter, I can't do too much of this cardio shit, or it'll hurt my strength."

Or would it?

Ramping Up Conditioning

As I continued getting older and learning that nobody gives a shit about how big or strong I am I eventually put my foot in the ground and said I am going to place as much emphasis on my conditioning as I do my strength training. If my size & strength go to hell, so be it, at least I'll be healthier.

This was around the same time I was at my wits end from destroying myself with the iron for so many years.

My hips hurt too bad to run or sprint, so I had to find other methods.

I started to dust off my old Prowlers and drag sleds and just went to town on them. Pushing, pulling, dragging, climbing stairs, skipping rope, doing farmers walks, & flipping tires. I was actually conditioning.

It felt damn good to do it, too.

And to my surprise, my strength didn't suffer, it improved. My work capacity improved. I could do *more* work, while experiencing *less* fatigue. I didn't hurt as bad. I started sleeping better. Damn near everything in my life got better when I started to prioritize conditioning.

Sure, I may have lost my "peak size and (weight room) strength" whatever the hell that means anyway, but for a young business owner with a young family who is focused on longevity and living (relatively) pain free, this conditioning stuff I ignored for so long because of an irrational fear of losing what I thought I cared about was the solution to the majority of my problems and I didn't even know it.

While you definitely have to account for conditioning in your training as it can certainly impede upon your recovery and have negative implications on your strength gains, I think many "weight room junkies" have a false perception of conditioning. I know I did.

Many people don't understand just how much it can help not only your overall health and preparedness levels, but your time in the weight room as well. A lot of lifters' limiting factors aren't their hamstrings or their triceps. It's their subpar work capacity that is limiting their progress.

Chapter 8:

Conditioning 101

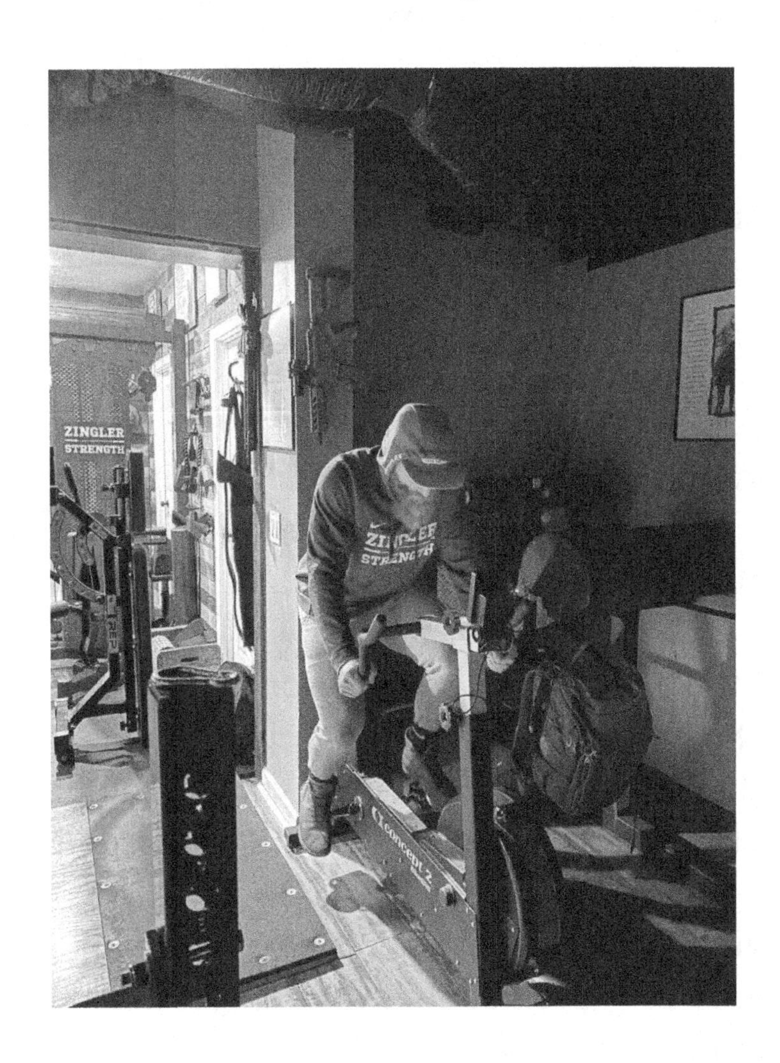

Conditioning is a simple concept. It's been made confusing over the last couple of decades by the egos of S&C Hardo's who have tried and succeeded at creating problems for every solution.

"Is it like steady state cardio? Or is it like the sleds and big tires? I thought conditioning was what they did before the football season?"

The answer is yes to all of the above.

To simplify, though, we will refer to 'ol Webster.

"Conditioning is the process of training to become physically fit by a regimen of exercise, diet, and rest."

That's it.

While there are certainly different types of conditioning, in a nutshell, conditioning is the process of becoming better prepared for the demands of life, training, sport, etc.

My goal is not to write a complex conditioning manual, outlining all of the science behind the different types of conditioning. As much as I am interested in the physiology behind it all, you probably aren't. If you are, check the resources list at the end of this book and dive in.

My goal is to give you actionable, applicable information that can help you improve your GPP levels so that you can get the most out of this system and improve your quality of life.

As I said in the strength section of this book, there is no one size fits all program, especially conditioning program.

It's very difficult to give specific conditioning programming guidelines to people with varying conditioning levels and goals because there are a wide variety of factors making it all but impossible to do so. These factors range from current fitness level, to injury history, to the type of surface you're pushing a sled on, if you even have access to a sled. Programming conditioning is not as simple as programming 3x5 @ 75% on Squats.

It would be ridiculous of me to say that somebody couldn't perform this program because they weren't initially fit enough to perform my interpretation of *hard* conditioning. It would also be unfair to limit someone's outputs with a prescribed set/rep/weight/range for a conditioning activity if their initial conditioning level is beyond my programmed recommendation.

While I will include sample templates and guidelines, it will serve you far better to teach you the simple conditioning concepts of this system.

This will allow you to build a program for *you*. Trying to do what I do, or he does may not always be what's best for you. Your training is about you, not them.

The theme of this system is simplicity, so if you guessed the conditioning aspect was going to be complex, you'd have guessed wrong.

Easy, Medium, Hard

Two of the biggest influences on the way I approach conditioning are Jim Wendler & Joel Jamieson. Joel is the author of the book 'Ultimate MMA Conditioning' which I believe to be one of the best books ever written on the subject of conditioning.

Jim Wendler, a very simple man himself, when explaining conditioning talks about it in two contexts:

Easy Conditioning & **Hard** Conditioning.

Complex Huh!?

Easy Conditioning - think walking.

Hard Conditioning - think pushing a heavy sled.

I've added the term: Medium Conditioning – think in the middle of the above two.

To give you the Ray Zingler explanation of Easy, Medium, & Hard Conditioning, here is what we're talking about:

Easy: Non-Taxing. A walk in the park.

Medium: Requires effort, but if you're with a friend, you can still maintain a conversation. I don't like training with people, but maybe you do.

Hard: Taxing, rigorous, effort requiring work. Your heart is pumping and the only conversation you're wanting to have is with yourself, very likely using foul language asking yourself why the hell you're doing this.

Sure, I can give you target heart rate ranges (see below) and all that jazz, but Easy, Medium, and Hard are pretty self-explanatory.

There are a variety of different interpretations for ideal heart rate ranges, but generally speaking, Easy Conditioning will fall in the 50%-70% Max HR Zone, Medium Conditioning will fall in the 70%-80% Max HR Zone, & Hard Conditioning will be north of 80% (for most).

To estimate your Maximum Heart Rate, the classic 220 – (minus) your age, works fine for most, but depending on your age, current fitness level, & overall health, this number can fluctuate.

Example: For a 25-year-old, their estimated Max HR would be 220 – 25 = 195.

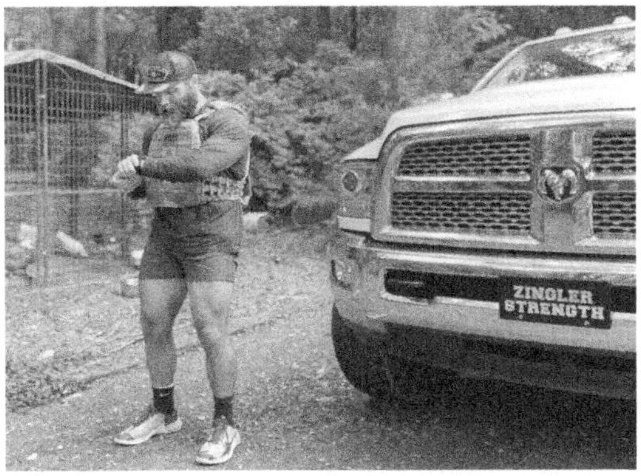

*Per the disclaimer in the beginning, please consult with your doctor if you have any questions or concerns regarding your specific target Heart Rate ranges.

The majority of the conditioning in this system calls for Easy and Medium Conditioning, however I do like to sprinkle in some Hard Conditioning in the form of Sleds, Intervals, Repeats, and Circuits once a week or so, but I assure you the Hard Conditioning isn't necessary.

I would argue that the Easy and Medium Conditioning is essential. These *types* of conditioning not only improve your overall health and well-being, they improve efficiency and the quality of your Strength sessions. Easy and Medium Conditioning also play a positive role in enhancing your recovery. Training is not about what you can do sometimes, it is about what you can consistently recover from.

Chapter 9:

Programming

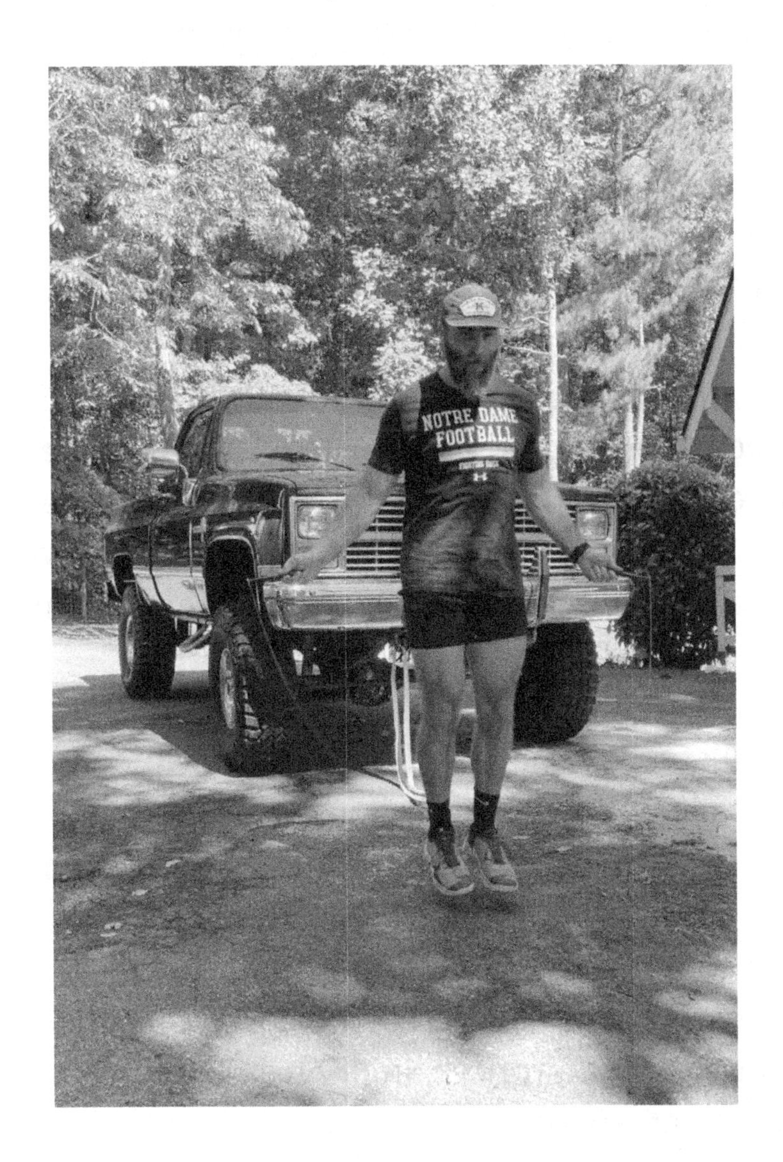

The most important conditioning principle I want you to take from this system is that there has to be a **goal**. There has to be a **why.**

You should never just go out and push a sled just to push it, flip a tire, to flip it, or jog an unknown distance just to jog.

Have a goal. It doesn't matter what that goal is, but have a goal. A short-term goal of what you want to do today and a long-term goal of what you want to be able to do a bunch of days from today.

This gives you purpose and something to aim at. Once you have purpose and a target, you simply reverse engineer your programming and set yourself up to progressively get to where you want to go.

If your short-term goal is to do 12 reps of 40 yards with 95 pounds on the Prowler today and your long-term goal is to do 16 reps of 60 yards with 135 pounds on it, go do your 12x40 with 95 today and progressively build week to week to attain your 16x60 with 135. It is a lot easier to maintain discipline when you can tangibly map out and see your progress.

The Prowler is just an example. This goes for any means of conditioning, Walking, Jogging, Rowing, Biking, it doesn't matter, you must have a goal. Doing it just to do it will always lead to stagnated progress.

I am first going to outline what I do and the tools I prefer to use and recommend, however there are a plethora of alternative options based on your conditioning preferences, injury history, current fitness level, access to equipment, space, time, etc.

The second most common question I get beyond the sets and reps questions from the strength section is "are there conditioning alternatives, if I don't have 'x'?" The answer is undoubtedly yes.

I realize most people have normal jobs and don't drive around town in a 2500 Ram 4x4 Truck with sleds and iron plates galore in the bed of it. You might not be able to go to an empty turf field in the middle of the day to train, so for you "normal" people, I will again first share how I designed the program and then provide some space/time saving alternatives.

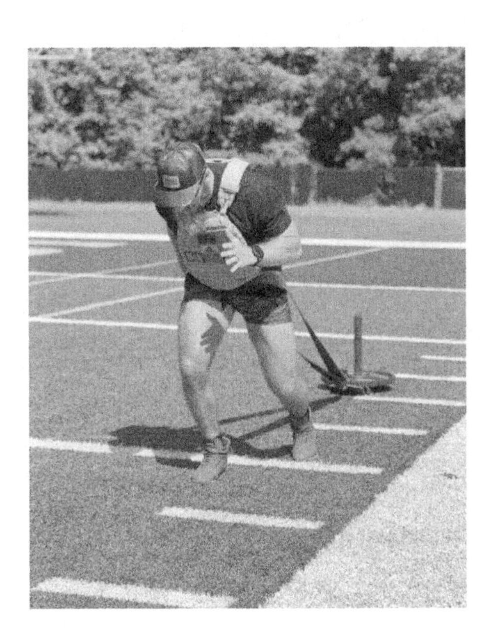

Template Options:

As outlined above, this program consists of Easy, Medium (required), and Hard (encouraged) Conditioning.

In some of the templates, the conditioning intensity progressively increases as the week progresses, however on the lower frequency templates, the *peak* conditioning day(s), might be midweek, on a Push/Pull Main Day, with easier conditioning prescribed on a Squat/Hinge Main Day.

Based on the template option you choose, I suggest programming the conditioning as follows: (Like the Strength section of the book, this section is only related to Conditioning). Your current fitness level will determine how you program conditioning intensities.

*Where you see "Strength & Conditioning" is just a simple reminder that if you choose that template option, you'll have Strength and Conditioning work on the same days. The "Easy, Medium, Hard" relates to the conditioning intensity, only.

6 Day

Day 1:
Day 2: Conditioning (Easy)
Day 3:
Day 4: Conditioning (Medium)
Day 5:
Day 6: Conditioning (Hard)

5 Day

Day 1:
Day 2: Conditioning (Easy)
Day 3:
Day 4:
Day 5: Conditioning (Medium/Hard)
Day 6: Strength & Conditioning (Easy)

4 Day

Day 1:
Day 2:
Day 3: Strength & Conditioning (Easy)
Day 4: Strength & Conditioning (Medium)
Day 5:

Day 6: Conditioning (Medium/Hard)

3 Day
Day 1: Strength & Conditioning (Easy)
Day 2: OFF
Day 3: Strength & Conditioning (Medium/Hard)
Day 4: OFF
Day 5: Strength & Conditioning (Easy)

2 Day
Day 1: OFF
Day 2: Strength & Conditioning (Medium/Hard)
Day 3: OFF
Day 4: Strength & Conditioning (Easy/Medium)

These are just templates, the most important part is simply committing to a template and getting the work in each week, how you go about it is far less important than simply getting it done.

Easy, Medium, & Hard Conditioning

While some conditioning modalities are obviously harder than others, for example, pushing a heavy Prowler is harder than walking around a track, it is very difficult to prescribe specific modalities as Easy, Medium, or Hard, simply because your current fitness level and the effort, intensity, weight, volume, etc. are going to be the major determinants of Easy, Medium, or Hard.

If I called sled dragging *Easy* and Prowler pushing *Hard*, but then told you to put 6 plates on the sled and drag it and push an empty Prowler, the Prowler is obviously easier than the Sled work.

This is why I say it's not about the tool, but the effort and intent.

I will now share which activities I personally choose for the Easy/Medium/Hard concepts. You are welcome to use these options or choose modalities that fit within the concepts.

Easy

For Easy days, I recommend:

- Walking
- Weight Vest Walking
- Light Rucking
- Light Sled Dragging (Forward & Backward)
- Jumping Rope
- Belt Squat Marching
- Stairs

Think of these as your "box checking" days. It's mundane, boring work. While your current conditioning level will drive what and how much you do, I typically recommend 20-60 minutes of any low-level activity of your choice. If you're *spent* after an easy conditioning day, you did it wrong.

*You can program as many Easy Conditioning sessions as you want per week. Most program templates call for 1-2, however, if it's possible to sneak micro easy sessions into your schedule via 10-minute daily walks or any low-level activity, I strongly encourage you to implement these as frequently as you can. Easy Conditioning is phenomenal for GPP development and mental health.

Summary:
- LOW level activity.
- 20-60 Minutes (1-2x/wk).
- As many 'micro' sessions as you'd like per week.

Medium

Medium Conditioning is really just an extension of Easy Conditioning, with a touch more kick. A lot of modalities I recommend are going to be the same with added intensity and increased effort.

For example, If I choose sled dragging as my Easy Conditioning choice, I'll likely use 1-2 plates on the sled and drag it 800-1,000 yards.

However, if I want to use the sled drag as my Medium Conditioning choice, I'll simply bump the weights to 3-4 plates on the sled & drag it 400-500 yards.

Sure, it's less overall volume, but the effort/work is increased, making this more of a *medium* choice. After a medium sled dragging session, I feel like I got in a great workout, but I am not by any means laying in the floor spent'

The reason I start with **sled dragging** is because it is my favorite Medium Conditioning tool.

For those who don't know what I am talking about, a simple drag sled is a small, inexpensive sled, with a single loadable post. You simply add weight (plates, sandbags, cinderblocks) to the sled, hook a strap up to it, and you then pull or drag it. There are a variety of other exercises that can be performed with the sled as well.

There are even cheap or free DIY sled options out there as well. Think rope and an old car tire.

The reason I like sled dragging so much is because it is very easy on the body. Sled dragging is largely concentric. While your legs and lungs will get a lot of quality work to improve your strength and conditioning, the sled will not leave you feeling beat up or sore.

I attribute my ability to train with such high frequency to the consistent use of the sled.

If the sled is something you can invest in and use, I would strongly encourage you to.

If the sled isn't an option, there are plenty of other modalities that can be used for your Medium Day(s).

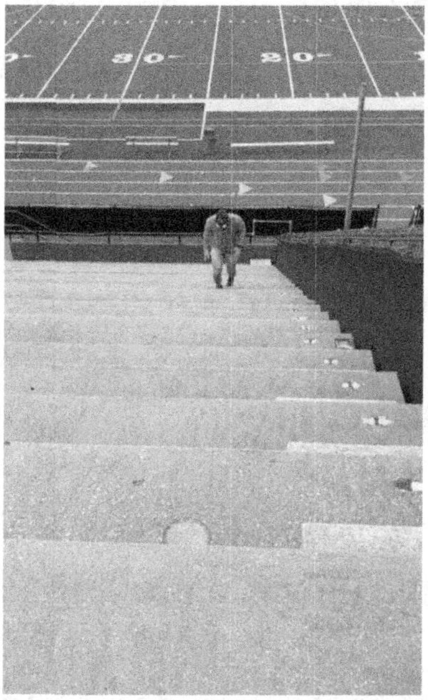

Some alternate options for Medium Days are:

1. Speed Walking
2. Running
3. Hiking
4. Prowler
5. Stair Walking
6. Stair Running
7. Hill Running
8. KB Complex
9. Light Carries
10. Bike, Rower, SkiErg, etc.

While this isn't an exhaustive list of your only Medium day options, simply pick what is feasible for you, and stay in that Medium range, erring closer to the Easy end than the Hard end.

Again, if Easy is a walk in the park and Hard is cussing yourself because 'this sucks', you're aiming in the middle, closer to Easy.

As far as *how much*? This is going to be entirely personal based on the variables consistently outlined in this manual.

I typically prefer to keep all Medium intensity sessions to around 20-40 minutes.

The key with Medium Conditioning, is again, not what you choose to do, but having a goal and progressive plan to improve accompanying it.

For example, let's say I choose sled dragging with 3 plates on it for my Medium day.

Here is an example of how I would program my Medium day's over a 4-week cycle:

Week 1: 10 x50 Yards w/ 3 Plates
Week 2: 12 x50 Yards w/ 3 Plates
Week 3: 15 x50 Yards w/ 3 Plates
Week 4 (Deload): 8x40 Yards w/ 2 Plates

*Plate = 45lbs. Plate

If you choose Running:

Week 1: 1.5 Mile Run
Week 2: 1.75 Mile Run
Week 3: 2 Mile Run
Week 4 (Deload): 1 Mile Run

If you choose Climbing Stairs:

Week 1: 20 Minutes of Stair Climbing
Week 2: 25 Minutes of Stair Climbing

Week 3: 30 Minutes of Stair Climbing
Week 4 (Deload): 15 Minutes of Stair Climbing

These are obviously very broad, bland examples and you would need to make your own informed modifications based on your current fitness level & personal variables, but just remember all conditioning needs to be goal oriented and progressive in nature.

If you don't have a goal at first, pick an activity that is a bit harder than a casual walk in the park and design it in a way that you know you can win. Next week, add a bit to it. The following week, add a bit more.

Just like with the strength work in this system, aim LOW and hit consistently. Don't try to hit a home run every time, singles win a lot of ball games. Remember consistency will always beat intensity.

There are a variety of ways to program Medium Conditioning, from manipulating rest periods, to adding distance to a run, or weight to a sled, but starting out remember to make your Medium closer to Easy.

Summary:
- Medium level activity.
- 20-40 Minutes (1-2x/week).
-Slowly increase outputs each week (shorter rest periods, reps, distance, weight, etc.).

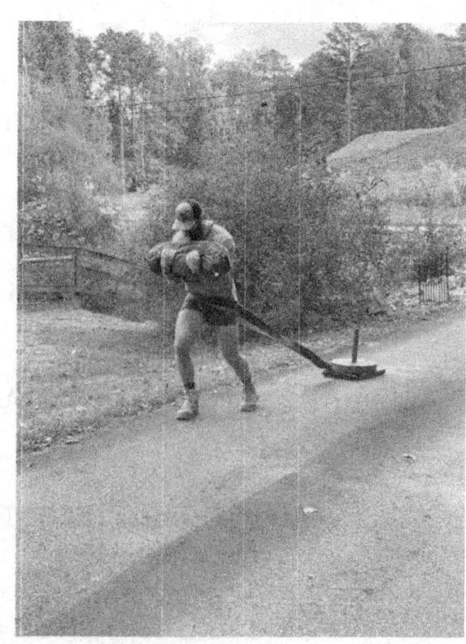

Hard

Hard Conditioning is not essential to this system; however I have found it to be valuable from a mental and physical challenge standpoint. I will share a story in the next chapter.

At the end of the day, this ENTIRE system is relative.

From your Main/Aux selections to your Easy, Medium, and Hard selections it is all relative to you.

My interpretation of Main and your interpretation of Main may be different.

Her interpretation of Medium may be different than his interpretation of Medium. The key with ALL of this stuff is that you run your race, not theirs.

For Hard Conditioning, personally speaking, I like to use the Prowler and other Anaerobic Conditioning methods, which, in layman's terms simply means *without oxygen*. These are going to be shorter, more intense bouts of exercise.

For Easy/Medium Conditioning, think **Low(er) Intensity & Long(er) Duration** to describe the majority of the work. For Hard Conditioning think **High(er) Intensity & Short(er) Duration** to describe the majority of the work.

The Prowler. Much like the sled, the Prowler is a great choice because while it is a son of a bitch, it is very simple to use and is easy on the body, in the sense that it's reasonable use will not leave you feeling sore, injured, and/or beat up the next day.

The Prowler is a man or (wo)man maker. As simple as the tool is, a triangular sled with two loadable plate posts on it, it is in my opinion the single best conditioning tool. It's simple, effective, and nearly impossible to mess up. I recommend the original Prowler from Elitefts.

I could write a dissertation on the Prowler, but I will spare you. If you have access to a Prowler or the funds to purchase one (or one like it) I strongly encourage you to use/get one.

You're probably picking up on the recurring theme of the impossibility of programming conditioning for a wide range of people, but this is especially true for the Prowler (and the sled) because it will move wildly differently (or not at all) depending on the surface you use it on (grass, turf, concrete, asphalt, etc.). Then you must factor in weather conditions on top of it.

If you have never pushed the Prowler, I would advise you to keep it very light and push it a short distance at first.

It's a very deceptive tool. It doesn't matter if you walk or run with it. It still sucks. You'll have a tendency to feel fine while you're pushing it, but the fatigue catches you when you finish.

To best program the Prowler it is best to push it on the same surface in similar conditions, if possible. If Week 1, you push it on turf, but week 2 you have to push it on grass, you will HAVE to adjust the weights used.

Example Program:

Week 1: 10x40 Yards w/ 95lbs
Week 2: 10x40 Yards w/ 115lbs.
Week 3: 10x40 Yards w/ 135lbs.

From this base template (whatever your base template is), you can begin to adjust variables: weight, distance, or rest periods, based on how you respond.

An unwritten rule of the Prowler, and most conditioning modalities is this: only adjust one (1) variable per workout (Credit: Jim Wendler).

Adding weight and distance will likely leave you miserable. Same can be said for shortening rest periods and adding distance. Learn how your body responds to the Prowler and then make informed programming decisions.

This does NOT need to be hypercomplex. Just progressive. Micro progressions lead to massive progress over time. Remember, this entire system is designed to help you win the long game.

Intervals, Repeats, & Circuits

As noted in the beginning of this section, my favorite book written on conditioning is 'Ultimate MMA Conditioning' by Joel Jamieson. If you're looking to take a deeper dive on the intricates of conditioning & energy system development, I strongly encourage you to pick up Joel's work.

The 3 Anaerobic Conditioning methods I like to use in this system (Outlined in Joel's book) are:

1) **Anaerobic (Lactic) Power Intervals**
2) **Anaerobic (Lactic) Explosive Repeats**
3) **Anaerobic (Lactic) Circuits**

Lactic Power Intervals

Lactic Power Intervals increase maximal HR and fast twitch power output.

I will explain how I program them, but the only important information is the durations of the sets/rest periods. The exercises can be anything you choose:

1. MedBall Slam 0:20 on 2:00 Rest x3 Rounds
2. 10 Min. Active Rest (Walk)
3. Bike Sprint 0:20 on 2:00 Rest x3 Rounds
4. 10 Min. Active Rest (Walk)
5. KB Swing 0:20 on 2:00 Rest x3 Rounds

You'll notice the reps last :20, I'm resting 2 minutes between sets, 10 minutes between *series*, performing 3 rounds per series, and 3 series per workout.

General guidelines for the Lactic Power Intervals: 20-40s per rep, 1-3 minutes rest between sets, 8-15 minutes rest between series, 3 reps per series, 2-4 series per workout.

Again, my exercises: MB Slams, Bike Sprint, and KB Swings are irrelevant. You can program any exercises you want, as long as you stay within the confines of the Work:Rest prescriptions.

You could choose Sprints, Box Jumps, and Shadow Boxing. It doesn't matter.

Then, to 'wave' (progress) this workout next week, and the week after, simply increase one (1) of the variables.

This could be adding an additional round, increasing work times, or decreasing rest times.

If you've never trained like this before, don't try to be a hero. Aim low and WIN. Then up the ante.

Lactic Explosive Repeats

The goal of Lactic Explosive Repeats is to improve lactic power and capacity as well as fast twitch power output.

Much like the Lactic Power Intervals, the durations are all you need to pay attention to, the exercises are unimportant.
An example of how repeats can be programmed are as follows:

1. :15 MB Slam x :30 Rest x 6 Rounds
2. 6 Min Active Rest (intermittent walking/skip rope/etc.)
3. :15 Treadmill/Outdoor Sprint x :30 Rest x 6 Rounds
4. 6 Min Active Rest (Intermittent walking/skip rope/etc.)
5. :15 lying MB No Throw x :30 Rest x 6 Rounds

You'll notice where repeats differ from intervals is the Work:Rest ratios. The work times are shorter, but so are the recovery periods.

General guidelines for Lactic Explosive Repeats: 1-3 *series* of 6-10 sets (rounds) for 1-3 exercises per workout. 6-8 minutes of active rest in between series.

If you choose to use this method, the key again is not the exercise selection, but the effort.

You'll want to increase your work times and decrease rest times each week.

3-week cycle example:

Week 1: 15s Work : 30s Rest
Week 2: 20s Work : 25s Rest

Week 3: 25s Work : 20s Rest

Note: This method breaks the *adjust one variable* rule and is NOT for the faint of heart. It is some of the hardest work I've ever done.

Anaerobic Lactic Circuits

Circuits are a simple, highly customizable option making them very popular. You've likely at least heard of or performed circuits of some sort.

The goal of Anaerobic (lactic) Conditioning Circuits is to develop lactic power and capacity.

You've picked up on the theme by now. Don't pay attention to the exercises, only the durations/rest periods, as the exercises can be of your choosing.

An example of how I program circuits is as follows:

1a. Jump Rope x :20
1b. SkiErg Sprint x :20
1c. BikeErg Sprint x :20
Rest – 2 Min.

-Repeat above set 3x thru.
-Active Rest 8-10 after the set.
-Repeat Above Circuit once more (twice total)

General guidelines for Anaerobic Lactic Circuits: :20-:30 per exercise, total duration of circuit should be 1-2 minutes, rest 1-3 minutes between circuit reps, perform 2-4 circuits per workout, resting 6-10 minutes between series.

If you were to use this base example as your week 1, to *wave* the intensity each week, you'd simply want to adjust a variable.

Increase work time, decrease rest time, add a circuit, etc. As long as you live within the duration/rest guidelines, how you progress a circuit is totally up to you.

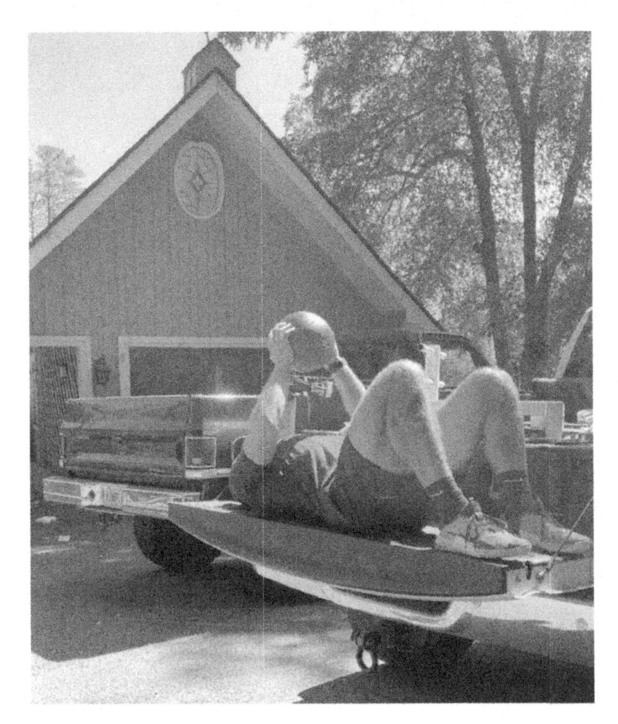

Hard Conditioning is Hard Conditioning. You can get as analytical and technical as you want, or you can pick up a rock in your back yard and run up hill with it. As long as it's Hard and you can progress the training session from week to week, it counts.

The idea isn't to beat the shit out of yourself, but whatever you choose, (if you choose to do Hard Conditioning), should be hard. Your heart rate should be elevated and you should be breathing heavy. This isn't a stroll in the mall, window shopping for cute outfits to wear to the local fitness center while you play on your phone. This is work.

That said, don't be an idiot. Make it hard, but set it up in a way you can progress each week. Aimlessly pushing yourself to the brink of exhaustion and calling it Hard Conditioning isn't progressive. It's stupid. Anybody can make themselves really tired. Making yourself better takes some common sense.

A few example modalities that you can use in addition to the outlined methods are:

1) Sprints
2) Hill Sprints
3) KB Complexes
4) BB Complexes
5) Bike Sprints
6) Rower Sprints
7) SkiErg Sprints
8) Heavier Sled Work
9) Medicine Ball Work
10) Stairs

Summary:
- High Intensity Activity.
- 15-40 Minutes (1x-2x sessions/wk.)
- Slowly increase outputs/manipulate variables each week.

Reminder: When planning your training, use duration, rest periods, rounds, reps, weights, etc. as your main variables to manipulate. Don't forget, it's always best to manipulate only 1 variable at a time. Though I have discussed many different conditioning activities, I will provide a final list of modalities you can choose from.

Conditioning Examples:

1) Sled
2) Prowler
3) Walking
4) Stairs
5) Sprints
6) Hills
7) Jump Rope
8) Kettlebells
9) Medballs
10) Weight Vest
11) Running/Walking
12) Rucking
13) Hiking
14) Lightweight Carries
15) Tire/Sledgehammer
16) Belt Squat Marching
17) Bodyweight Calisthenics
18) SkiErg
19) Bike
20) Rower
21) Additional indoor Cardio Equipment

Chapter 10:

135 Pound Prowler. 1,000 Yards. 30 Minutes.

– My Misogi.

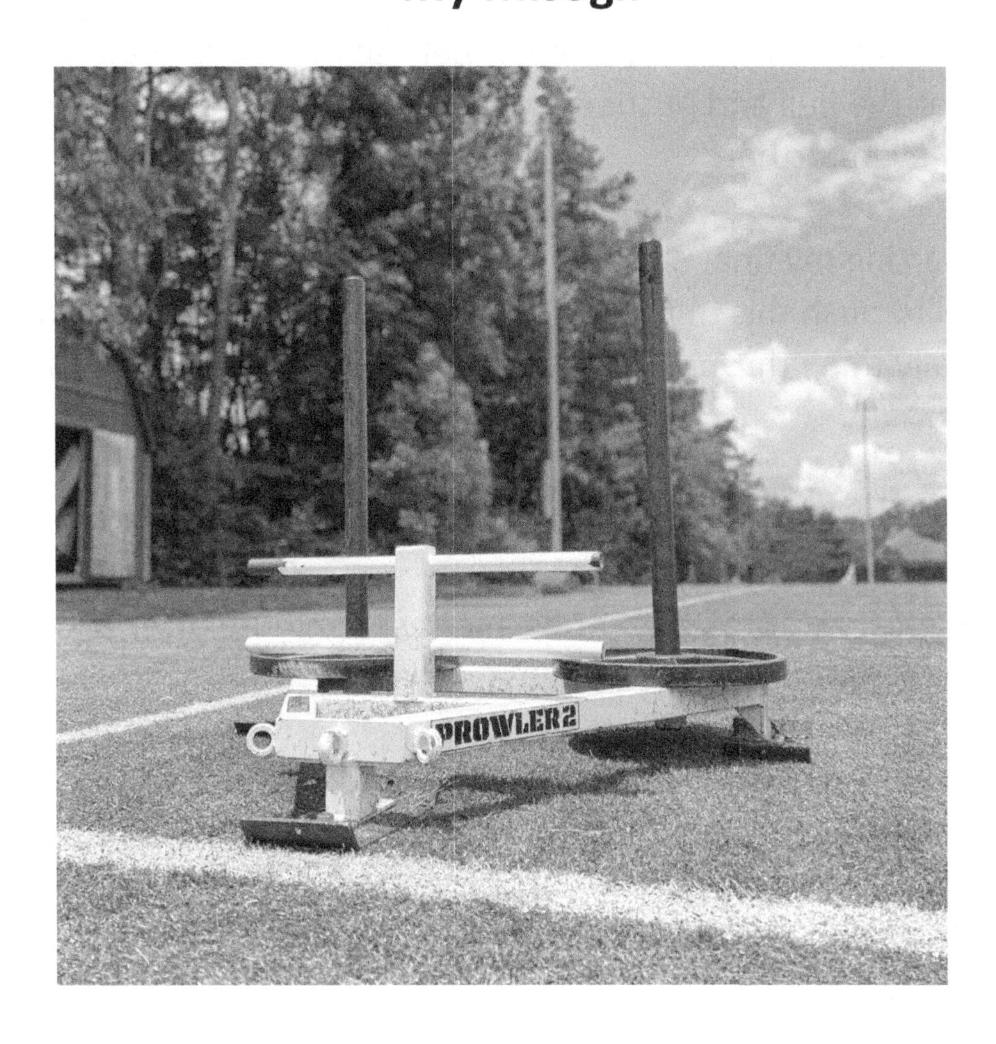

Back in the Spring of 2022, I was out pushing the Prowler at the local high school.

I had planned on pushing it for a half hour or so that day, but didn't really have any rules. I wasn't doing sets of a specific distance. I wasn't timing rest periods. I'd just push it the length of the field and turn it around and push it back. The *goal* was to push it for a half hour, so I just went to pushing.

At the end of that half hour, I remember feeling really good that day, so I said what the hell and pushed it a little further. Then a little further. And then even further.

Before starting my final trip back to the truck, I told myself, I'm going to set a goal to push this thing 1,000 yards in 30 minutes. At the moment, I didn't really think through the logistics. It just sounded good, so I rolled with it.

As I was driving home, I was doing the math in my head.

"If I push it 50 yards in 30 seconds and rest 1 minute after each rep, I just have to sustain that for 20 reps."

"Wait, what!?" This meathead guy is going to try to push 135-pound Prowler 50 yards x 20 reps with 60s rest in between each push?

Nah, nevermind that sounds crazy. Let's think of a more *realistic* goal.

"But, hmm, could I do it?"

This is when my Misogi was born.

A Misogi, a concept I learned about reading Michael Easter's fantastic book, 'The Comfort Crisis', (which I highly recommend by the way), is very simple.

It is a goal. A goal that has two simple rules.

1) Have a 50% or greater chance of failure.
2) Don't die.

That's it.

I wrestled back and forth about actually committing to the goal, because the more I played it out in my head, it just sounded insane. It may not be for you, but it is a bit farfetched for a guy like me.

Eventually I committed to the goal and went all in.

I had an idea of where I was at, but wanted to get a better idea so I could create a training plan to at least give myself a chance to reach this goal.

I went out the following week and pushed it just under 800 yards in 30 minutes.

I wasn't *testing* myself yet, per se, because again, I wasn't allowed to die, but really just gauging where I was.

Week after week, I would drag that Prowler out & push it. I was wearing HR Monitors, fancy watches, tracking all the data, experimenting with different distances per set, you name it, I was trying it.

One day nearing summer, after a consistent stretch of fairly easy sessions of 12x50 yard pushes in my *target interval range* (30s work:1 minute rest), I decided it was time to test myself.

On my first test day, I pushed The Prowler 900 yards in 30 minutes.

Only 100 yards away from my goal! So close!

There was only one problem.

I nearly broke rule number 2 of my Misogi, don't die.

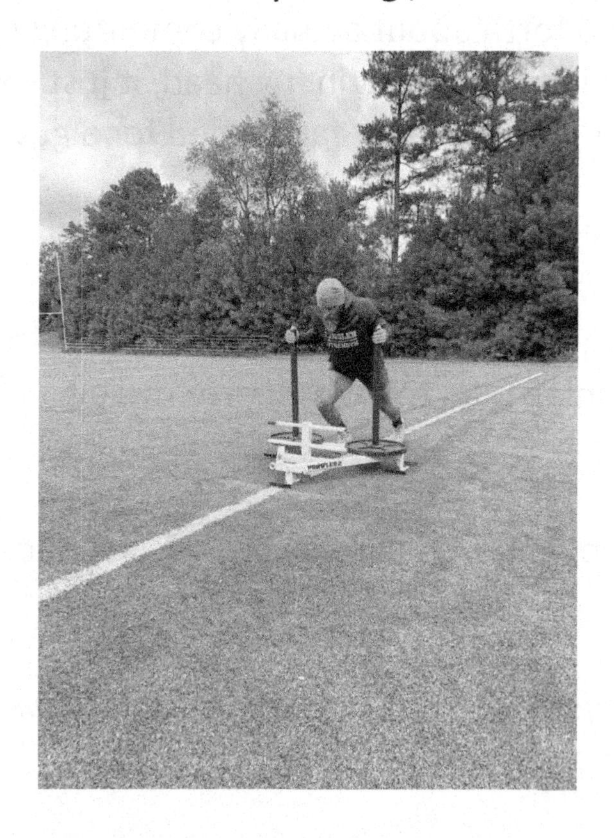

When I tell you I gave damn near everything I had to finish the 900th yard in 30 minutes, I gave it everything I had.

I was seeing all the stars. I was dizzy. I couldn't get my breathing under control. I was beyond spent and thought Jesus was taking me home.

After finally getting my breathing under control and stabilizing my heart rate (my Garmin watch thought I was dying). I cleaned up my Prowler and drove home, encouraged, but confused.

I really want to do it, I think it's possible, but how the hell am I going to squeeze out these extra 100 yards, when 900 nearly took me to the Pearly Gates?

I went back to the drawing board.

I added an additional day of Prowler work to my training. I programmed a light weight (95lbs) & long (80+ yards) day and a heavy (185lbs+) & short (<50 yards) day.

I kept my head down week in and week out, and relentlessly attacked my Prowler training, harder than I've ever attacked any training in my life.

I wasn't sure if it was possible, but I was damn determined to accomplish the feat.

About 6 weeks from my 900-yard PR, I had the Prowler out during a deload week.

I set the timer for 30 minutes and was planning to push it no more than 4-500 yards or so. The plan was to push it my normal protocol, 50 yards (30s) and rest 1 minute for a few reps and then rest a few minutes before performing another few 50-yard bouts.

Again, this was a deload (recovery) week, so I certainly wasn't trying to do anything too taxing.

I turned on some music and got started.

The first 50-yard trip went like butter. So did the second. The third and fourth too.

Again, I was planning on resting a bit after 3-4 50-yard trips, but for whatever reason I was feeling it that day. It may have been the Hank Williams Jr. blasting in my earbuds, but who knows. Onward I went.

I was waiting for that normal HR Spike I'd get around the 12th or so rep, but I never got it. And holy shit, I'm not on pace, I'm ahead of schedule.

I felt like I could push the Prowler forever on that day.

However, knowing that fatigue could catch me at any time, I intentionally slowed myself down and got back close to pace.

But today was the day, I don't know why, it wasn't planned, (I was planning on attempting the test again, near my birthday on August 15) I had no intentions of accomplishing it, but it was crushed.

I achieved my goal. I smoked my Misogi. 135 Pound Prowler, 1000 yards, in 29 minutes.

I was happy. For about 10 seconds.

My mindset didn't shift to mad after those 10 seconds, but more like "well no shit it happened, I worked for that."

I loaded up my Prowler, went home, and ate some lunch.

3 days later, I drug the Prowler back out and pushed it again, following the protocol I had planned for the next Prowler session.

It was never really about *the goal*. It was always and still is about the process.

Why Having a Goal is Important

I'm not telling you to attempt the 1,000 Yard Prowler Challenge. I'm not even telling you to do Hard Conditioning.

135 pounds on your sled might feel like 50 pounds or 350 pounds depending on the surface you're pushing it on. You may not even have a Prowler and that's fine.

My goal(s) don't need to be your goals. They need to be yours and they need to matter to you.

While I've intentionally been repetitive in this book to drive home certain points, the one concept I've stressed more than any other is to have a goal.

The reason having goals is so important is because goals make your process mean something.

If you don't have a goal at first, you have to define your *why.* Are you doing this for you? For your spouse? So you can be around to watch your children grow up? Why? Once you have a why, you can create a goal. And that *why* behind your goal will be the driving force of your discipline & personal accountability.

Something happens in your mind as you start chipping away and getting closer to what you've set out to accomplish.

It took me several months from that early Spring day when I committed to the challenge to accomplishing it on that late July morning.

Looking back on it I see just how valuable that goal was. That goal forced me to be intentional about every training session. I knew that without relentless, committed effort, I had no chance.

It upped the ante not only on my Prowler days, but my strength training sessions, my sled dragging sessions, my weight vest walks. My sleeping habits. That goal made it all matter just a little bit more.

That goal was accomplished in 29 minutes, a shorter length of time than the average Netflix Show.

But the months of relentless effort leading up to those 29 minutes was where the real value was. Each and every time I went out to prepare to achieve my goal, I was casting votes for the more committed person I wanted to be, the more resilient person I wanted to be, the more disciplined person I wanted to be.

The process is where all the fruit is.

Make sure you have goal. It'll pay you.

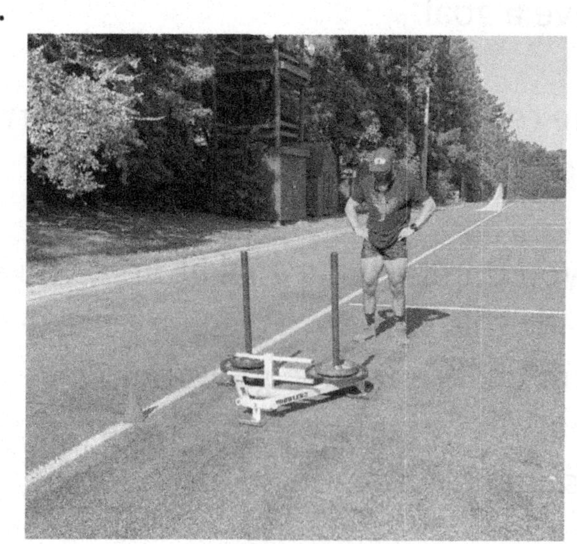

Chapter 11
Conditioning Wrap Up:

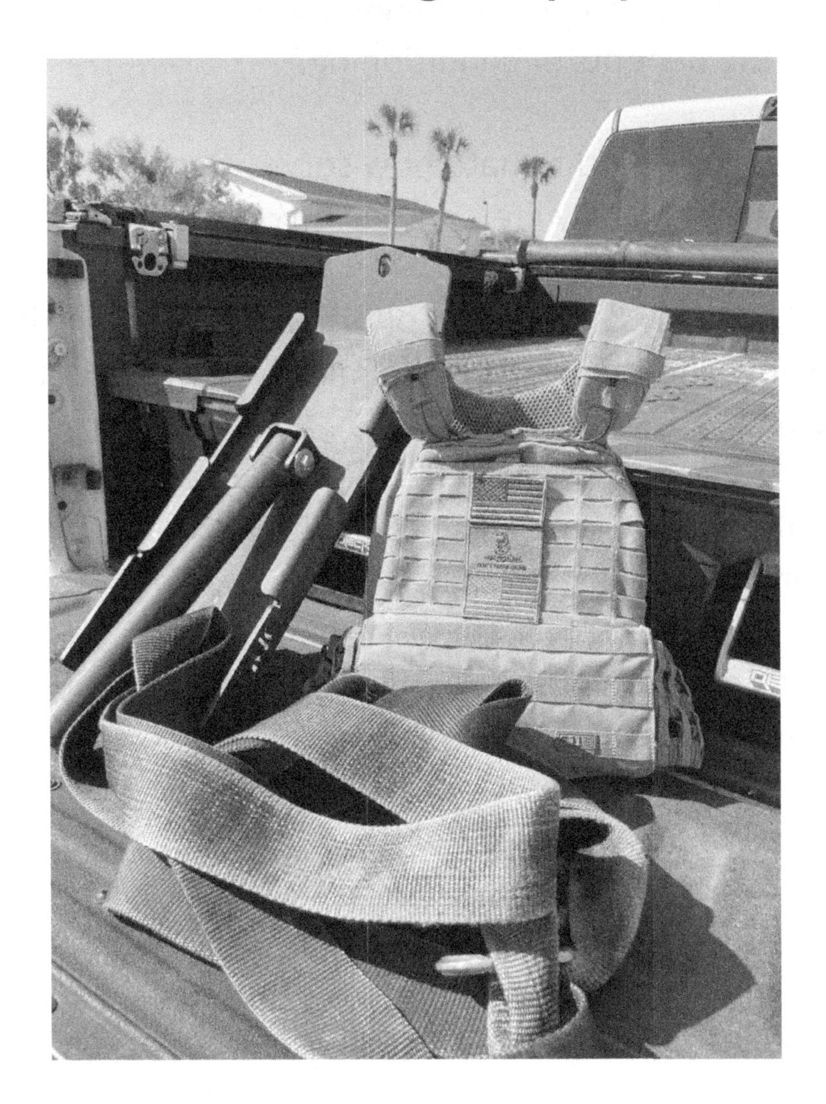

Conditioning doesn't have to be complex. In fact, it shouldn't be. By suppressing complexity, you free up bandwidth for sound execution.

Over the years as I have progressively increased my focus on conditioning, I've watched my quality of life improve.

I've also noticed that I don't even have to do *that much* or go *that hard* to really reap the benefits of conditioning.

Conditioning which I used to hate now serves as one of the most therapeutic activities in my life.

I cut my teeth on Easy & Medium Conditioning and sprinkle in hard bouts every now and then. This is the mindset I would encourage you to have as well.

It doesn't matter what you choose to do, it only matters that you do it with intentionality and consistency.

To summarize Conditioning:

Step 1:
Honestly assess where you are at with your current fitness level.

Step 2:
Have a plan and be goal oriented. It doesn't matter what your plan or goal is, you just have to have one to prevent aimless activity and stagnated progress.

Step 3:
Start easy. Go slow. Set yourself up to win. Check boxes.

Step 4:

Make sure what you're doing is progressive. Modestly adjust your variables (1 at a time). Slow and steady progression is the way.

Step 5:

Stay consistent. The best way to never have to get ready is to always stay ready.

**Micro Easy Conditioning sessions are valuable. Simple 10–20-minute walks sprinkled into your week have an immense amount of value.

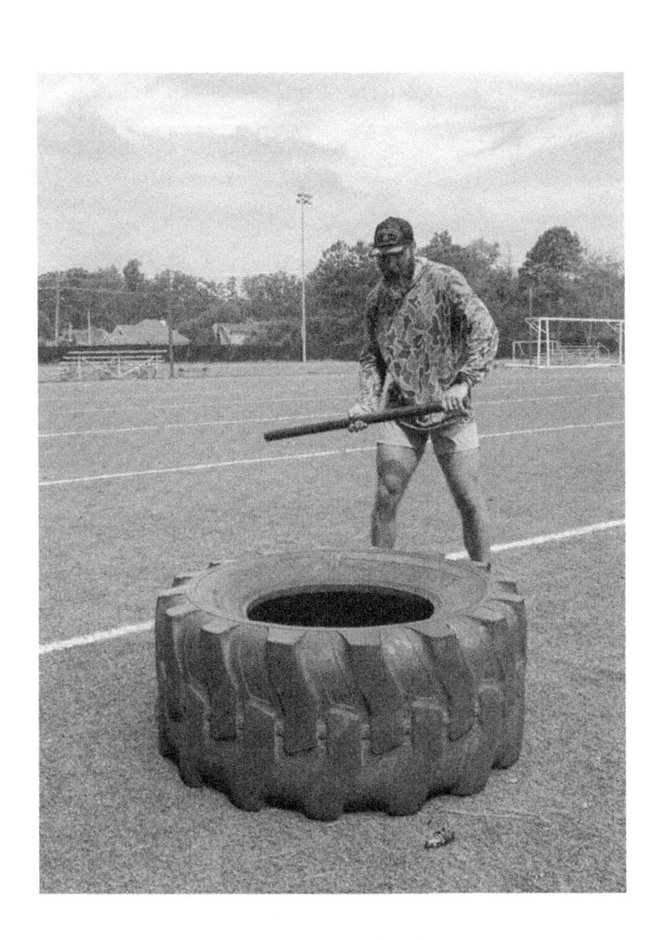

Section 3:

Diet, Supplements, & Recovery

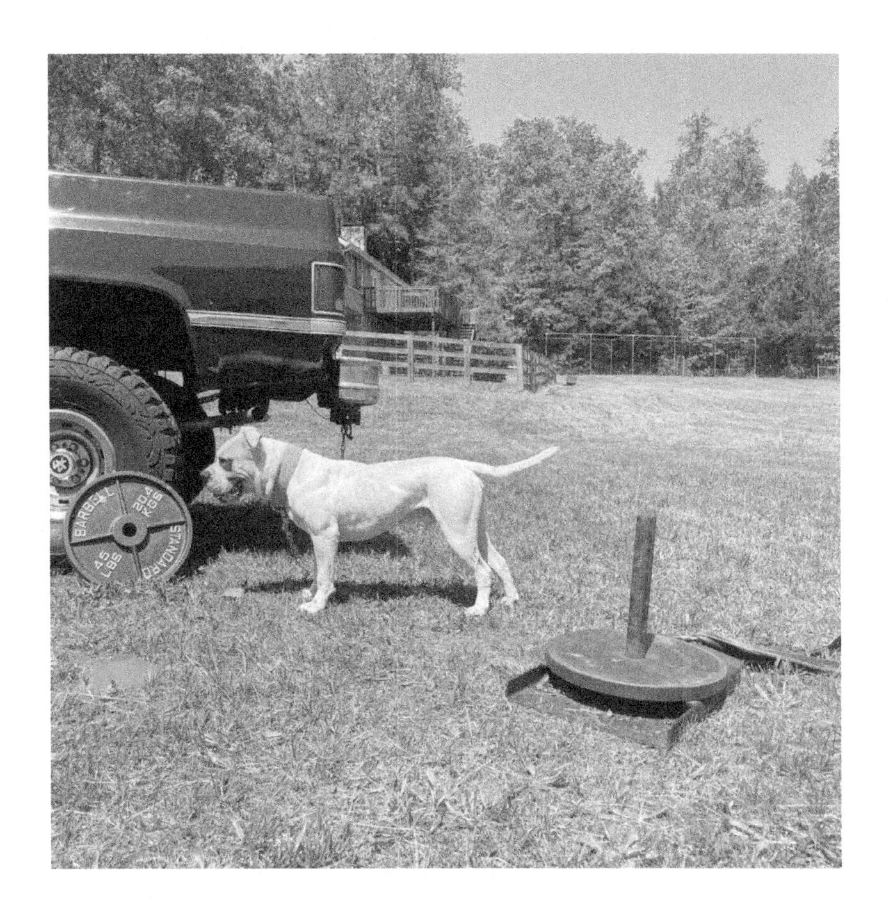

Chapter 12:

Diet

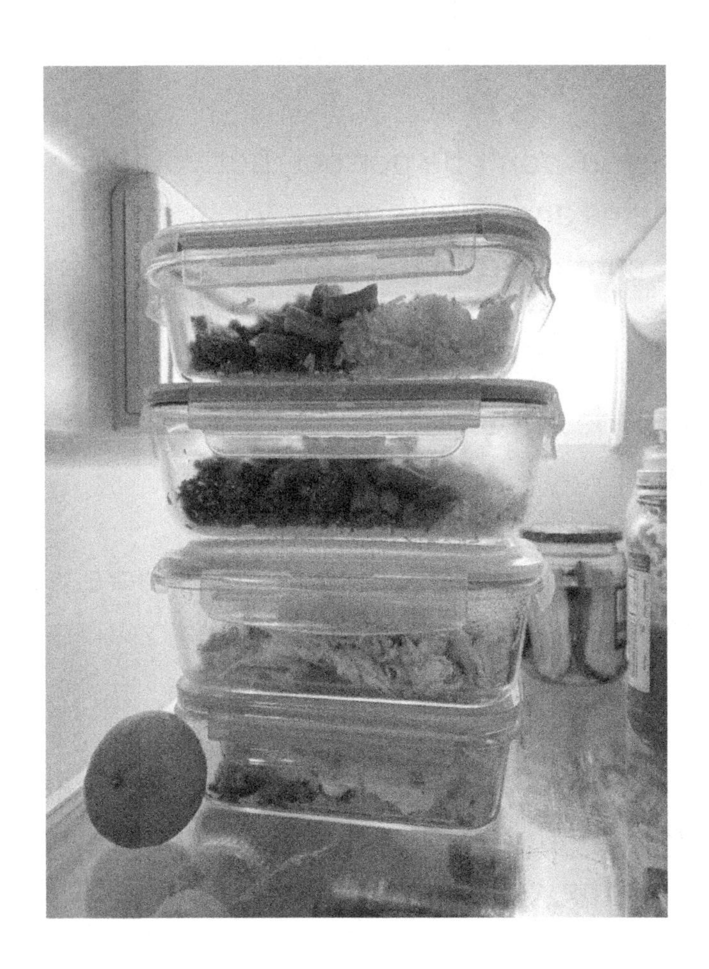

This is going to be the shortest section of this book because there are a plethora of resources on the topic.

There are a million different diets out there and truth be told, most of them work provided you consistently hold up to your end of the deal. A lot of people seem to miss that little caveat.

I heed Dan John's advice here:
"Eat Like an Adult."

If you can do this, you won't be perfect, but you'll reduce the likelihood of potential problems and you'll solve a lot of existing ones. Rest assured, this isn't coming from the mountain top. I eat pizza and burgers, too.

As far as your diet goes, you need to eat and drink in a way that reflects your desires/goals.

If you're looking to gain weight, you'll need to increase your calories, ensuring you stay in a caloric surplus, meaning you eat more calories than you burn.

If you're looking to lose weight, you'll need to decrease your calories, but still eat enough to fuel your body, aiming to stay in a sustainable caloric deficit, meaning, you burn more calories that you eat.

If you can't/don't eat in a way that will help you attain your goals, you care more about staying where you are than you do making progress.

Cutting edge advice, huh? But truthfully that is all there is to it.

Do what works for you. If it doesn't work for you, change or modify.

If intermittent fasting works for you, intermittent fast. If Weight Watchers works for you, do Weight Watchers. Regardless of what you choose to do, nothing will ever be more important than consistency. Notice I didn't say, perfection, but consistency.

I have a rule for myself that I can't say will work for everyone, but it works for me:

"Don't eat like an asshole most of the time." This allows me to eat like an asshole sometimes.

Personally speaking, I like principles from Stan Efferdings 'Vertical Diet', but I largely believe in eating a balanced diet full of Protein, Complex Carbohydrates, and Healthy Fats.

Find what works for you & stick to it the majority of the time.

Chapter 13:

Supplements

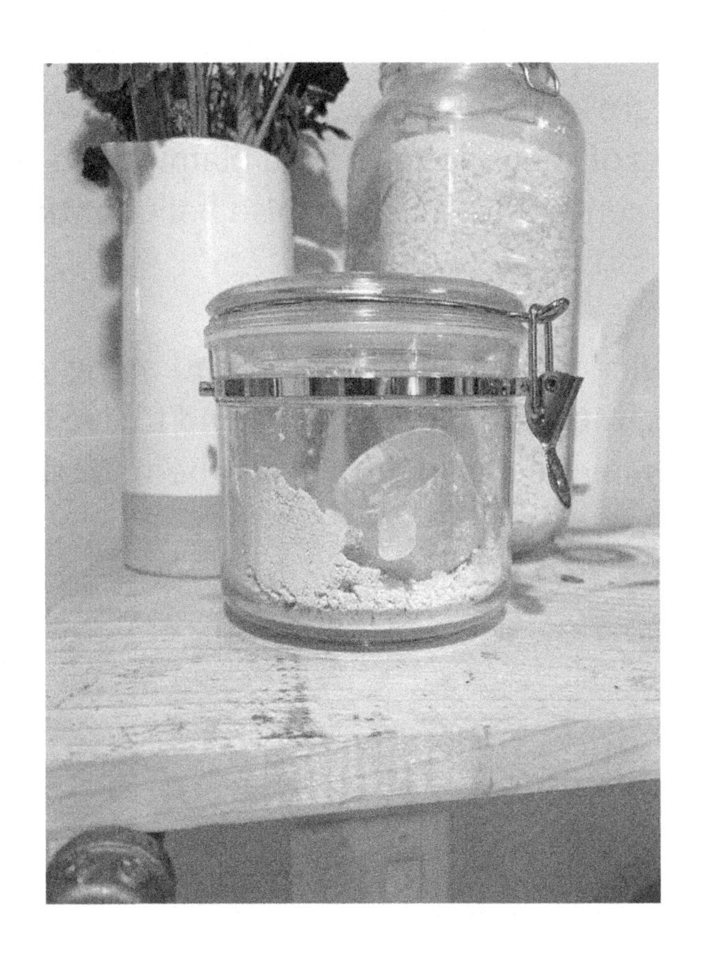

I've taken every supplement under the sun. Some work, some don't. However, the MOST important thing to understand about supplements is this: A supplement is intended to SUPPLEMENT your diet, not replace anything in your diet.

I see too many High School kids who have the latest & greatest pre workout and post workout drinks, but eat like rabbits and wonder why they struggle to make progress.

It's because they are attempting to use supplements to replace essential elements of their diet and then blaming the supplements for not working. This contributes to their false belief of themselves being "hard gainers."

While I am not giving medical advice or encouraging you to take or not take supplements, the supplements that tend to live in my daily diet are typically vitamin/mineral based, but I'll list them for those interested.

-Vitamin B Complex
-Vitamin C
-Vitamin D
-VitaminK2
-Glucosamine & Chondroitin
-Creatine Monohydrate
-Turmeric
-Psyllium Fiber
-Beef Liver
-Electrolytes
-L-Carnitine
-L-Theanine
-Low Dose Melatonin
-Low Dose ZMA

I always buy the highest quality supplements that I can find.

If you want to drink protein shakes, pre-workout, and all that stuff, that's fine. Make sure the supplements you choose to take are researched and high quality. Regardless of what you choose to take, remember supplements are only intended to supplement your diet. If you're using supplements to replace or skip anything, save your money for food, or whatever else, because you won't get out of supplements what you think you will if the foundation of your diet is not based in whole food nutrition.

Consult your doctor before taking any supplements. Don't listen to me.

Chapter 14:

Recovery

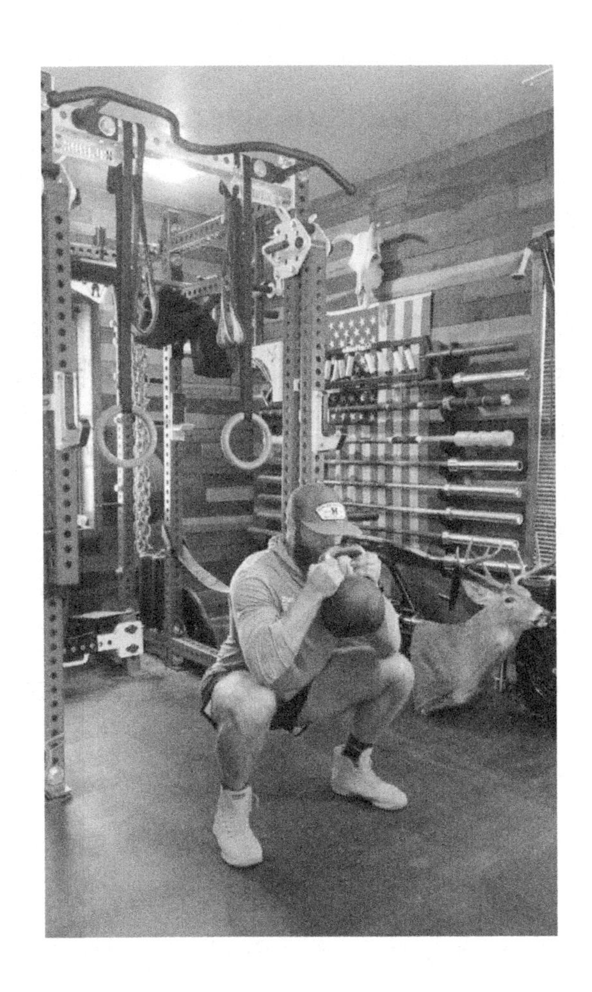

Foam Rollers, Massage Guns, Compression Boots. I have used all that stuff. They work fine, however nothing works better than eating, resting, and hydrating properly.

We briefly touched on diet in the previous chapter, so I will spend a little time talking on some fundamentals of rest and hydration.

Rest

While obviously getting 7-8 hours of sleep is pretty much common knowledge these days (there are personal variances to the range), I am going to go with a bit of a non-traditional angle on sleep.

If you're not getting adequate rest because you're choosing to stay up late playing video games, watching Netflix, or TikTok, then that's on you. Turn the screen off and go to sleep.

However, I know there are many people out there who would love to get 7-8 hours of sleep a night, but they have trouble getting to sleep, staying asleep, or waking in the middle of the night. Many people in the world suffer from sleep disturbances for a variety of reasons, me included.

I used to use all of these sleep trackers from watches to bands, to rings, and etc. I've used all of them to *predict* my day's readiness. While I'm not saying those devices are entirely garbage, they would essentially accentuate my stress levels related to my desire to get quality sleep. The stress from wanting to sleep well lead to further increased disturbances. Not fun.

So, Step 1 if you're not sleeping well, do away with all the trackers. They add insult to injury.

Beyond that a few things that I like to do to increase the quality of my sleep are as follows:

1) Set the thermostat to 65-68 degrees.
2) Use a fan, more for the noise, than the wind in your face.
3) Sleep in a pitch black room with comfortable bedding and pillow(s).
4) Go to bed and wake up at the same time, every day. Weekends included.
5) Get some sort of movement and outdoor light exposure within 30 minutes of waking up.
6) Always drink 16oz. of water before any caffeine.
7) Strategically dose sun exposure throughout the day.
8) Never over caffeinate, but definitely cut caffeine by 3pm.
9) Do not train too late in the evening. My preferred time to train is midday/afternoon.
10) Do not eat a large meal too close to bedtime.
11) Perform Breathwork before bed to activate the parasympathetic nervous system. I like the “Box Breathing” app created by Mark Divine.
12) Read a fiction novel before bed.

*If I do have a bad night's sleep, I try not to let it get the best of me. I typically combat my poor night's sleep with increased water intake, increased sun exposure, and increased levels of low-level activity.

Again, my sleep recommendations are not medical advice, they are just things that have helped improve my sleep quality over the years.

Hydration

Working with youth athletes for a living, I am constantly preaching the importance of hydration and it typically falls on deaf ears until that one cramp hits them. The physical cue is one of the best lessons to teach anyone to prioritize hydration.

Hydration is for the most part a controllable. Water isn't too expensive and plastic bottles aren't either. Thank God for modern conveniences. All you have to do is simply drink it.

Sure there are recommendations of ½ gallon, to a gallon, to two gallons depending on where you look, but I think ½ gallon a day is a good starting point for most people.

If you sweat more, you'll need to increase your fluid intake to replace the heightened levels of lost fluids.

A caveat to drinking water, though, is that you don't just want to drink copious amounts of purified water, especially if you're sweating a lot. As I assume you know, when you're sweating your body is releasing a lot more than simply water.

Chugging a whole bunch of purified water to rehydrate yourself is only going to make you urinate more. It isn't going to replenish the electrolytes your body lost. (Note electrolytes in my daily supplement regimen.) If you don't have/want to use an electrolyte supplement, simply add a few dashes of high-quality sea salt to your water. You won't taste it, but you will replenish some of what you lost through sweating.

Again, I am a S&C Coach, not a doctor or nutritionist, take the advice at face value.

Lastly, this program, while high(er) in frequency, is submaximal & low(er) in volume by design. This was designed intentionally to make the work performed highly recoverable. This design element was extremely important to me because I'm learning that as I get older, I'm rarely operating at my *100% of my best.* But even if I'm only feeling *okay,* hell even less than okay, I can still punch the clock and win the day.

These workouts should not leave you feeling beat down into the ground. If they are, re-read the book.

If you're following the templates as they are laid out and are progressing slowly, you shouldn't need to use any extravagant recovery methods.

The rest days and Easy Conditioning days will build your work capacity and enhance your recovery.

As always, if there are any certain recovery methods you enjoy utilizing, use them.

Conclusion

This isn't just a system I threw together in 3 days. This has been a product of years and years of study, trial, and error.

This system has gaps in it, every system ever written does. This system is not the only way. Hell, I'm not even saying it's the best way. It's just a way that I have found works.

While I have laid out template examples for you to follow, you can customize your Broad Axe Training any way you want using the Squat, Hinge, Push, Pull, Carry, Easy, Medium, & (optional) Hard Conditioning.

Regardless of how you set it up, the most important elements are frequency and consistency.

Have a plan, stick to the plan, but if you get off track, simply get back on.

The best cowboys are not the most talented ones, but the ones who consistently get back on the horse.

Life happens. You will get sick, you will have to go out of town, and that 'thing' will come up out of nowhere. It happens to us all.

The unique thing about this program is that the patterns can be performed anywhere, with anything, regardless of how you're feeling or what life throws at you.

For example, let's say you come down with a nasty cold right before a heavy week of training. It'd probably be wise NOT to do a bunch of heavy squats and deadlifts, right?

But can you still Squat, Hinge, Push, Pull, and Carry? Can you do some Easy Conditioning? Hell yeah you can.

A few sets of easy Bodyweight Squats, DB RDLs, Push Ups, Bodyweight Rows, and Light Dumbbell carries, coupled with some low intensity walks in the sunshine is phenomenal *down week* prescription.

As much as I'd love to always stick to the plan, I've regularly called audibles and performed training weeks that look exactly like the above. Is it perfect? No. Does it keep me consistent and moving forward? You bet your ass.

If you have a down week, whether it's controllable or not, simply adjust and stay in the fight.

My hope is that I've at least laid the groundwork for you to develop a very simple Strength & Conditioning Program that allows you to make consistent progression over long periods of time.

You may love the concepts or hate the concepts, but my hope is that at the very least you were able to take something from them.

While the end of this book lays out 12-Week template examples (the minimum amount of time I would encourage you to run this system), you can run this type of training for as long as you would like to.

There are an endless variety of ways to Squat, Hinge, Push, Pull, Carry & perform Easy, Medium, and Hard Conditioning.

Thank you for taking the time to read up on The Broad Axe System, it is a culmination of the continued evolution of my life's work and I hope you benefit from it.

I wish you the best and must leave you with this:

Do not overthink. Just do the work. Then repeat it. Consistency always wins.

In Strength,

Ray Zingler

Section 4:

Template Examples

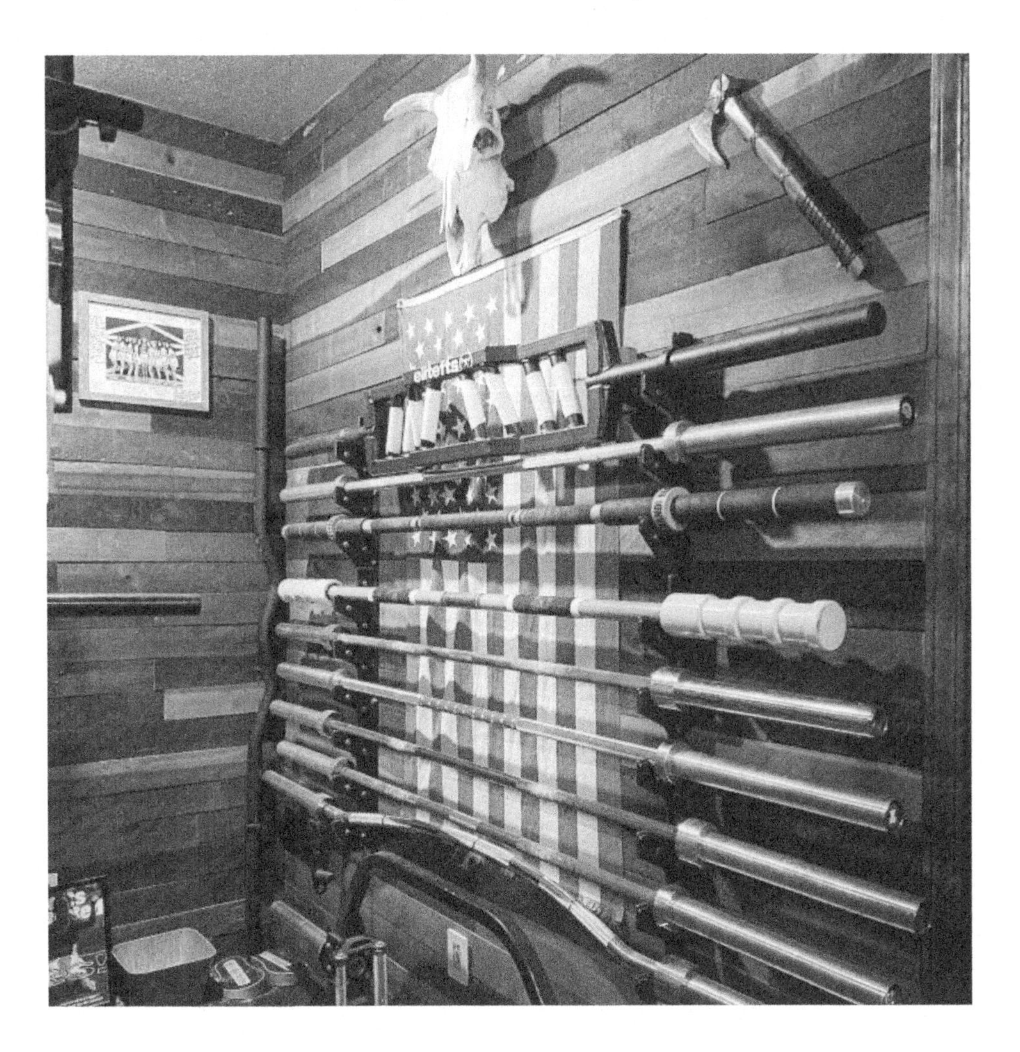

Template Example Options:

6 Day

Day 1: Strength (Aux Focus on All Lifts)
Day 2: Conditioning (Easy)
Day 3: Strength (Squat/Push Main, Hinge/Pull Aux)
Day 4: Conditioning (Medium)
Day 5: Strength (Hinge/Pull Main, Squat/Push Aux)
Day 6: Conditioning (Hard)

5 Day

Day 1: Strength (Squat Main, Hinge/Push/Pull Aux)
Day 2: Conditioning (Medium)
Day 3: OFF
Day 4: Strength (Push/Pull Main, Squat/Hinge Aux)
Day 5: Conditioning (Hard)
Day 6: Strength & Conditioning (Hinge Main, Squat/Push/Pull Aux & Easy Cond.)
Day 7: OFF

4 Day

Day 1: Strength (Squat Main, Hinge/Push/Pull Aux)
Day 2: OFF
Day 3: Strength & Conditioning (Push/Pull Main, Squat/Hinge Aux & Med. Cond.)
Day 4: Strength & Conditioning (Hinge Main, Squat/Push/Pull Aux & Easy Cond.)
Day 5: Off
Day 6: Conditioning (Hard Conditioning)

3 Day

Day 1: Strength & Conditioning (Squat Main, Hinge/Push/Pull/Aux & Med. Cond.)
Day 2: OFF
Day 3: Strength & Conditioning (Push/Pull Main, Squat/Hinge Aux & Heavy Cond.)
Day 4: OFF
Day 5: Strength & Conditioning (Hinge Main, Squat/Push/Pull Aux & Light Cond.)

2 Day

Day 1: OFF
Day 2: Strength & Conditioning (Squat/Press Main, Hinge/Pull Aux & Light/Med Cond.)
Day 3: OFF
Day 4: Strength & Conditioning (Hinge/Pull Main, Squat/Push Aux & Med Cond.)

Depending on the Template you choose, you might have to modify your *outputs*. The higher frequency templates allow you to spread your workload over the majority of the days of the week, where the lower frequency templates will require you to combine your Strength & Conditioning training on the same day. Because of the lower volume nature of the program, you shouldn't have too much issue combining S&C together, but it is something you should account for.

Each of the 12-Week templates provided are nothing more than **Examples.** Of course, you can follow them, but you're welcome to plug and play from the exercise lists provided.

Choose exercises that will help you reach your goals.

Do you want to improve barbell strength? Program a lot of barbell work and then choose Aux Exercises that will enhance the lifts you're looking to improve.

Are you looking to improve your strength, but your main focus is conditioning, running specifically? Program lighter DB/KB exercises on your strength days and cut your teeth with a variety of running workouts during the week.

You can set it up however you want. Maybe AM Conditioning and PM Strength Training works for you? Vice Versa?

Maybe you work 24 hours on and 48 hours off so you need to create your own template?

You travel several weeks a month & don't have access to 'x' when you're away? There are dumbbells in every hotel gym. Go Squat, Hinge, Push, Pull, & Carry them. Climb stairs at the hotel.

Don't be afraid to try and experiment with your own ideas. Keep what works for you and scrap what doesn't.

I will lay out a 12 Week/6-Day Template, a 12 Week/3-Day Template, and a 12 Week/3-Day *Minimalist* Template so you can see exactly how I would write up a program.

You'll notice for example purposes; I adjust the exercise selections for all lifts every 4 weeks (at the start of a new cycle). Remember, if you're a beginner, this may not be a good idea, especially if you're using the 5/3/1 Percentage Protocol to program your weights. Run YOUR program.

If you choose a 5,4-, or 2-Day Template simply use the guides provided and build your program based on the training frequency option you choose.

Can you perform the following training cycles exactly as they're written? Maybe. Maybe not. Use them as a guide and adapt where needed.

Start out easy and set yourself up to win the long game.

12-Week/6-Day Training Template

6 Day/Week 1

Day 1: Strength (Aux Focus on all Lifts)

1. Belt Squat– 3x10
2. Barbell RDL – 3x10
3. Flat Bench DB Press – 3x10
4. Dumbbell Row – 3x10
5. KB Carry – 3x:30

Day 2: Conditioning (Easy)

1. Forward Sled Drag – 12x60 Yards 40% of BW on Sled

Day 3: Strength (Squat/Push Main, Hinge/Pull Aux)

1. Barbell Back Squat – 3x 5, 5, 5+
2. KB Swing – 3x10
3. Incline BB Bench Press – 3x 5, 5, 5+
4. Pull Up/BW Row – 3x10
5. Single Arm Suitcase Carry – 3x:30

Day 4: Conditioning (Medium)

1. Prowler Push w/ 1 plate/side – 500 Yards (10x50 Yards)

Day 5: Strength (Hinge/Pull Main, Squat/Push Aux)

1. KB Goblet Squat – 3x10
2. Trap Bar Deadlift – 3x 5, 5, 5+
3. Push Up – 3x10
4. Barbell Row – 3x 8, 8, 8
5. Odd Object Carry – 3x:30

Day 6: Conditioning (Hard -- Anaerobic Lactic Power Interval)

6. MedBall Slam 0:20 on 2:00 Rest x3 Rounds
7. 5-10 Min. Active Rest (Walk)
8. Bike Sprint 0:20 on 2:200 Rest x3 Rounds
9. 5-10 Min. Active Rest (Walk)
10. KB Swing 0:20 on 2:00 Rest x3 Rounds

Day 7: OFF/Active Rest

1. Totally OFF, Walking, Light Sled Dragging, Extra Mobility Work, etc. all acceptable here.

6 Day/Week 2

Day 1: Strength (Aux Focus on all Lifts)

1. Belt Squat– 4x10
2. Barbell RDL – 4x10
3. Flat Bench DB Press – 4x10
4. Dumbbell Row – 4x10
5. KB Carry: 3x:40

Day 2: Conditioning (Easy)

1. Forward Sled Drag – 12x60 Yards 50% of BW on Sled

Day 3: Strength (Squat/Push Main, Hinge/Pull Aux)

1. Barbell Back Squat – 3x 3, 3, 3+
2. KB Swing – 4x10
3. Incline BB Bench Press – 3x 3, 3, 3+
4. Pull Up/BW Row – 4x10
5. Single Arm Suitcase Carry : 3x:40

Day 4: Conditioning (Medium/Hard)

1. Prowler Push w/ 1 plate/side – 600 Yards (12x50 Yards)

Day 5: Strength (Hinge/Pull Main, Squat/Push Aux)

1. KB Goblet Squat – 4x10
2. Trap Bar Deadlift – 3x 3, 3, 3+
3. Push Up – 4x10
4. Barbell Row –3x 5, 5, 5+
5. Odd Object Carry – 3x:40

Day 6: Conditioning (Hard -- Anaerobic Lactic Power Interval)

1. MedBall Slam 0:20 on 2:00 Rest x4 Rounds
2. 5-10 Min. Active Rest (Walk)
3. Bike Sprint 0:20 on 2:00 Rest x4 Rounds
4. 5-10 Min. Active Rest (Walk)
5. KB Swing 0:20 on 2:00 Rest x4 Rounds

Day 7: OFF/Active Rest

1. Totally OFF, Walking, Light Sled Dragging, Extra Mobility Work, etc. all acceptable here.

6 Day/Week 3

Day 1: Strength (Aux Focus on all Lifts)

1. Belt Squat– 4x12
2. Barbell RDL – 4x12
3. Flat DB Press – 4x12
4. DB Row – 4x12
5. KB Carry: 3x:45

Day 2: Conditioning (Easy)

1. Forward Sled Drag – 12x60 Yards 60% of BW on Sled

Day 3: Strength (Squat/Push Main, Hinge/Pull Aux)

1. Barbell Back Squat – 3x 5,3,1+
2. KB Swing – 4x12
3. Incline BB Bench Press –3x 5, 3, 1+
4. Pull Up/BW Row – 4x12
5. Single Arm Suitcase Carry: 3x:45

Day 4: Conditioning (Medium/Hard)

1. Prowler Push w/ 1 plate/side – 750 Yards (15x50 Yards)

Day 5: Strength (Hinge/Pull Main, Squat/Push Aux)

1. KB Goblet Squat – 4x12
2. Trap Bar Deadlift – 3x 5, 3, 1+
3. Push Up – 5x10
4. Barbell Row – 4x 5, 5, 5, 5+
5. Odd Object Carry: 3x:45

Day 6: Conditioning (Hard -- Anaerobic Lactic Power Interval)

1. MedBall Slam 0:20 on 2:00 Rest x5 Rounds
2. 5-10 Min. Active Rest (Walk)
3. Bike Sprint 0:20 on 2:200 Rest x5 Rounds
4. 5-10 Min. Active Rest (Walk)
5. KB Swing 0:20 on 2:00 Rest x5 Rounds

Day 7: OFF/Active Rest

1. Totally OFF, Walking, Light Sled Dragging, Extra Mobility Work, etc. all acceptable here.

6 Day/Week 4 – Deload (Mains should be performed ~50-60% intensity)

Day 1: Strength (Aux Focus on all Lifts)

1. Belt Squat– 3x5
2. Barbell RDL – 3x5
3. Flat DB Press – 3x5
4. DB Row – 3x5
5. KB Carry: 3x:30

Day 2: Conditioning (Easy)

1. Forward Sled Drag – 10x60 Yards 40% of BW on Sled

Day 3: Strength (Squat/Push Main, Hinge/Pull Aux)

1. Barbell Back Squat – 3x5
2. KB Swing – 2x10
3. Incline BB Bench Press – 3x5
4. Pull Up/BW Row – 2x10
5. Single Arm Suitcase Carry: 3x:30

Day 4: Conditioning (Medium/Hard)

1. Prowler Push w/ 1 plate/side – 300 Yards (6x50 Yards)

Day 5: Strength (Hinge/Pull Main, Squat/Push Aux)

1. KB Goblet Squat – 2x10
2. Trap Bar Deadlift – 3x5
3. Push Up – 2x10
4. Barbell Row – 3x5
5. Odd Object Carry: 3x:30

Day 6: Conditioning (Hard --Anaerobic Lactic Power Interval)

1. MedBall Slam 0:20 on 2:00 Rest x2-3 Rounds
2. 5-10 Min. Active Rest (Walk)
3. Bike Sprint 0:20 on 2:200 Rest x2-3 Rounds
4. 5-10 Min. Active Rest (Walk)
5. KB Swing 0:20 on 2:00 Rest x2-3 Rounds

Day 7: OFF/Active Rest

1. Totally OFF, Walking, Light Sled Dragging, Extra Mobility Work, etc. all acceptable here.

6 Day/Week 5

Day 1: Strength (Aux Focus all Lifts)

1. Pause Belt Squat – 3x10
2. Single Leg DB RDL – 3x10 Ea. Leg
3. Incline DB Press – 3x10
4. KB Gorilla Row – 3x10
5. KB Goblet Carry – 3x:30

Day 2: Conditioning (Easy)

1. Reverse Sled Drag – 12x60 w/ 40% of BW on Sled

Day 3: Strength (Squat/Push Main, Hinge/Pull Aux)

1. Barbell Back Squat – 3x 5, 5, 5+
2. Barbell Glute Bridge – 3x10
3. Flat Barbell Bench Press – 3x 5, 5, 5+
4. TRX/Ring Row – 3x10
5. KB Front Rack Carry – 3x:30

Day 4: Conditioning (Medium/Hard)

1. Prowler Push – Increase weight from weeks 1-3, 500 yards (10x50 yards)

Day 5: Strength (Hinge/Pull Main, Squat/Push Aux)

1. KB Pause Goblet Squat – 3x10
2. Deficit Trap Bar Deadlift – 3x 5, 5, 5+
3. Decline Push Up – 3x10
4. Inverted Grip BB Row –3x 8, 8, 8+
5. Sandbag Carry – 3x:30

Day 6: Conditioning (Hard -- Anaerobic, Lactic Explosive Repeat)

6. :15 MB Slam x :30 Rest x 6 Rounds
7. 6 Min Active Rest (intermittent walking/skip rope/etc.)
8. :15 Treadmill/Outdoor Sprint x :30 Rest x 6 Rounds
9. 6 Min Active Rest (Intermittent walking/skip rope/etc.
10. :15 lying MB No Throw x :30 Rest x 6 Rounds

Day 7: OFF/Active Rest

1. Totally OFF, Walking, Light Sled Dragging, Extra Mobility Work, etc. all acceptable here.

6 Day/Week 6

Day 1: Strength (Aux Focus on all Lifts)

1. Belt Pause Box Squat – 4x10
2. Single Leg DB RDL – 4x10 Ea. Leg
3. Incline DB Press – 4x10
4. KB Gorilla Row – 4x10
5. KB Goblet Carry – 3x:40

Day 2: Conditioning (Easy/Medium)

1. Reverse Sled Drag – 12x60 w/ 50% of BW on Sled

Day 3: Strength (Squat/Push Main, Hinge/Pull Aux)

1. Barbell Back Squat – 3x 3, 3, 3+
2. Barbell Glute Bridge – 4x10
3. Flat Barbell Bench Press – 3x 3, 3, 3+
4. TRX/Ring Row – 4x10
5. KB Front Rack Carry – 3x:40

Day 4: Conditioning (Medium/Hard)

1. Prowler Push – Use same weight as last week, 600 yards – (10x60 yards)

Day 5: Strength (Hinge/Pull Main, Squat/Push Aux)

1. KB Pause Goblet Squat – 4x10
2. Deficit Trap Bar Deadlift – 3x 3, 3, 3+
3. Decline Push Up – 4x10
4. Inverted Grip BB Row – 3x 5, 5, 5+
5. Sandbag Carry – 3x:40

Day 6: Conditioning (Hard -- Anaerobic, Lactic Explosive Repeat)

1. :20 MB Slam x :25 Rest x 6 Rounds
2. 6-10 Min Active Rest (intermittent walking/skip rope/etc.)
3. :20 Treadmill/Outdoor Sprint x :25 Rest x 6 Rounds
4. 6 Min Active Rest (Intermittent walking/skip rope/etc.
5. :20 lying MB No Throw x :25 Rest x 6 Rounds

Day 7: OFF/Active Rest

1. Totally OFF, Walking, Light Sled Dragging, Extra Mobility Work, etc. all acceptable here.

6 Day/Week 7

Day 1: Strength (Aux Focus on all Lifts)

1. Belt Pause Box Squat– 4x12
2. Single Leg DB RDL – 4x12 Ea. Leg
3. Incline DB Press – 4x12
4. KB Gorilla Row – 4x12
5. KB Goblet Carry – 3x:45

Day 2: Conditioning (Easy/Medium)

1. Reverse Sled Drag – 12x60 w/ 60% of BW on Sled

Day 3: Strength (Squat/Push Main, Hinge/Pull Aux)

1. Barbell Back Squat – 3x 5,3,1+
2. Barbell Glute Bridge – 4x12
3. Flat Barbell Bench Press – 3x 5, 3, 1+
4. TRX/Ring Row – 4x12
5. KB Front Rack Carry – 3x:45

Day 4: Conditioning (Medium/Hard)

1. Prowler Push – Use same weight as last week, 750 yards – (15x50 yards)

Day 5: Strength (Hinge/Pull Main, Squat/Push Aux)

1. KB Pause Goblet Squat – 4x12
2. Deficit Trap Bar Deadlift – 3x 5, 3,1+
3. Decline Push Up – 4x12
4. Inverted Grip BB Row – 4x 5, 5, 5, 5+
5. Sandbag Carry – 3x:45

Day 6: Conditioning (Hard -- Anaerobic, Lactic Explosive Repeat)

1. :25 MB Slam x :20 Rest x 6 Rounds
2. 6 Min Active Rest (intermittent walking/skip rope/etc.)
3. :25 Treadmill/Outdoor Sprint x :20 Rest x 6 Rounds
4. 6 Min Active Rest (Intermittent walking/skip rope/etc.
5. :25 lying MB No Throw x :20 Rest x 6 Rounds

Day 7: OFF/Active Rest

1. Totally OFF, Walking, Light Sled Dragging, Extra Mobility Work, etc. all acceptable here.

6 Day/Week 8 – Deload (Mains should be performed ~50-60% intensity)

Day 1: Strength (Aux Focus on all Lifts)

1. Belt Pause Box Squat/Pause Front Squat – 3x5
2. Single Leg DB RDL – 3x5 Ea. Leg
3. Incline DB Press – 3x5
4. KB Gorilla Row – 3x5
5. KB Goblet Carry – 3x:30

Day 2: Conditioning (Easy/Medium)

1. Reverse Sled Drag – 10x60 w/ 50-60% of BW on Sled

Day 3: Strength (Squat/Push Main, Hinge/Pull Aux)

1. Barbell Back Squat – 3x5
2. Barbell Glute Bridge – 2x10
3. Flat Barbell Bench Press – 3x5
4. TRX/Ring Row – 2x10
5. KB Front Rack Carry – 3x:30

Day 4: Conditioning (Medium/Hard)

1. Prowler Push – 1 plate/side, 500 yards (5x50 yards)

Day 5: Strength (Hinge/Pull Main, Squat/Push Aux)

1. KB Pause Goblet Squat – 2x10
2. Deficit Trap Bar Deadlift – 3x5
3. Decline Push Up – 2x10
4. Inverted Grip BB Row – 3x5
5. Sandbag Carry – 3x30

Day 6: Conditioning (Hard -- Anaerobic, Lactic Explosive Repeat)

1. :15 MB Slam x :30 Rest x 3 Rounds
2. 6 Min Active Rest (intermittent walking/skip rope/etc.)
3. :15 Treadmill/Outdoor Sprint x :30 Rest x 3 Rounds
4. 6 Min Active Rest (Intermittent walking/skip rope/etc.
5. :15 lying MB No Throw x :30 Rest x 3 Rounds

Day 7: OFF/Active Rest

1. Totally OFF, Walking, Light Sled Dragging, Extra Mobility Work, etc. all acceptable here.

6 Day/Week 9

Day 1: Strength (Aux Focus on all Lifts)

1. Sandbag Squat – 3x10
2. Banded Pull Through – 3x10 Ea. Leg
3. DB Floor Press – 3x10
4. Lat Pulldown– 3x10
5. Bottoms Up KB Carry – 3x:30

Day 2: Conditioning (Easy)

1. Forward Sled Drag – 6x60 yards w/ 65% of BW on Sled
2. Reverse Sled Drag – 6x60 yards w/ 65% of BW on Sled

Day 3: Strength (Squat/Push Main, Hinge/Pull Aux)

1. Safety Squat Bar Squat – 3x 5, 5, 5+
2. KB Good Morning – 3x10
3. Barbell Overhead Press– 3x 5, 5, 5+
4. Band Face Pull – 3x10
5. KB Single Arm Carry – 3x:30

Day 4: Conditioning (Medium/Hard)

1. Prowler Push – Increase weight from weeks 4-6, 600 yards (12x50 yards)

Day 5: Strength (Hinge/Pull Main, Squat/Push Aux)

1. Front Rack KB Goblet Squat – 3x10
2. Straight Bar Deadlift – 3x 3, 3, 3+
3. Pause Push Up (in bottom) – 3x10
4. Pendlay Row– 3x 8, 8, 8+
5. Heavy Rock/MB Carry – 3x:30

Day 6: Conditioning (Hard -- Anaerobic (Lactic) Conditioning Circuit Training Method)

1a. Jump Rope x :20
1b. SkiErg Sprint x :20
1c. BikeErg Sprint x :20
Rest – 2 Min.

Repeat above cluster 2x thru
Active Rest 8-10 after the "set"

Repeat Above Circuit once more (twice total)

Day 7: OFF/Active Rest:

1. Totally OFF, Walking, Light Sled Dragging, Extra Mobility Work, etc. all acceptable here.

6 Day/Week 10

Day 1: Strength (Aux Focus on all Lifts)

1. Sandbag Squat– 4x10
2. Banded Pull Through – 4x10 Ea. Leg
3. DB Floor Press – 4x10
4. Lat Pulldown – 4x10
5. Bottoms Up KB Carry – 3x:40

Day 2: Conditioning (Easy/Medium)

1. Forward Sled Drag – 6x60 w/ 75% of BW on Sled
2. Reverse Sled Drag – 6x60 w/ 75% of BW on Sled

Day 3: Strength (Squat/Push Main, Hinge/Pull Aux)

1. Safety Squat Bar Squat – 3x 3, 3, 3+
2. KB Good Morning – 4x10
3. Barbell Overhead Press – 3x 3, 3, 3+
4. Band Face Pull – 4x10
5. KB Single Arm Carry – 3x:40

Day 4: Conditioning (Medium/Hard)

1. Prowler Push – Use same weight as last week, 700 yards – (14x50 yards)

Day 5: Strength (Hinge/Pull Main, Squat/Push Aux)

1. Front Rack KB Goblet Squat– 4x10
2. Straight Bar Deadlift – 3x 3, 3, 3+
3. Pause Push Up (in bottom) – 4x10
4. Pendlay Row – 3x 5, 5, 5+
5. Heavy Rock/MB Carry – 3x:40

Day 6: Conditioning (Hard -- Anaerobic (Lactic) Conditioning Circuit Training Method)

1a. Jump Rope x :20
1b. SkiErg Sprint x :20
1c. BikeErg Sprint x :20
Rest – 2 Min.

Repeat above cluster 3x thru
Active Rest 8-10 min after the "set"

Repeat Above Circuit once more (twice total)

Day 7: OFF/Active Rest:

1. Totally OFF, Walking, Light Sled Dragging, Extra Mobility Work, etc. all acceptable here.

6 Day/Week 11

Day 1: Strength (Aux Focus all Lifts)

1. Sandbag Squat– 4x12
2. Banded Pull Through– 4x12 Ea. Leg
3. DB Floor Press– 4x12
4. Lat Pulldown – 4x12
5. Bottoms Up KB Carry– 3x:45

Day 2: Conditioning (Easy)

1. Forward Sled Drag – 6x60 yards w/ 85% of BW on Sled
2. Reverse Sled Drag – 6x60 yards w/ 85% of BW on Sled

Day 3: Strength (Squat/Push Main, Hinge/Pull Aux)

1. Safety Squat Bar Squat – 3x 5,3,1+
2. KB Good Morning – 4x12
3. Barbell Overhead Press – 3x 5, 3, 1+
4. Band Face Pull – 4x12
5. KB Single Arm Carry – 3x:45

Day 4: Conditioning (Medium/Hard)

1. Prowler Push – Use same weight as last week, 800 yards – (16x50 yards)

Day 5: Strength (Hinge/Pull Main, Squat/Push Aux)

1. Front Rack KB Goblet Squat– 4x12
2. Straight Bar Deadlift– 3x 5, 3, 1+
3. Pause Push Up (in bottom) – 4x12
4. Pendlay Row – 4x 5, 5, 5, 5+
5. Big Rock/Heavy MB Carry – 3x:45

Day 6: Conditioning (Hard -- Anaerobic (Lactic) Conditioning Circuit Training Method)

1a. Jump Rope x :25
1b. SkiErg Sprint x :25
1c. BikeErg Sprint x :25
Rest – 2 Min.

Repeat above cluster 4x thru
Active Rest 8-10 min after the "set"

Repeat Above Circuit once more (twice total)

Day 7: OFF/Active Rest:

1. Totally OFF, Walking, Light Sled Dragging, Extra Mobility Work, etc. all acceptable here.

6 Day/Week 12

You have 3 options here.

Option 1:
Deload the previous 3-week cycle, in similar fashion that you deloaded weeks 1-3 & 5-8's cycle & then start a new cycle the following week. (Week 13)

Option 2:
If you're feeling good, go ahead & program another 3-week cycle using the outline exemplified in weeks 1-11.

Option 3:
If you have any Personal Record (PR) Goals, whether they be 1RM's, Rep Maxes, or Conditioning Challenges, feel free to use this week to test yourself. After a testing week, you may deload, start a new 3-week cycle, or do what you wish with your training.

12-Week/3-Day Training Template

3 Day/Week 1

Day 1: S&C (Squat Main, Hinge/Push/Pull Aux + Easy Conditioning)

1. Barbell Back Squat – 3x 5, 5, 5+
2. KB Swing – 3x10
3. Incline DB Bench Press – 3x10
4. Pull Up/BW Row – 3x10
5. Single Arm Suitcase Carry – 3x:30
6. Forward Sled Drag – 12 x 50 Yards w/ 35% of BW

Day 2: S&C (Push/Pull Main, Squat/Hinge Aux + Medium Conditioning)

1. DB Bulgarian Split Squat – 3x10
2. DB RDL – 3x10
3. Barbell Bench Press – 3x 5, 5, 5+
4. T-Bar Row – 3x 8, 8, 8+
5. Sandbag Carry – 3x:30
6. Stairs – x20 Minutes

Day 3: S&C (Hinge Main, Squat, Push, Pull Aux + Easy Conditioning)

1. Goblet Squat - 3x10
2. Conventional Deadlift – 3x 5, 5, 5+
3. Overhead DB Press – 3x10
4. DB Row – 3x10
5. Trap Bar Carry – 3x:30
6. Weight Vest Walk – x20 Minutes

3 Day/Week 2

Day 1: S&C (Squat Main, Hinge/Push/Pull Aux + Easy Conditioning)

1. Barbell Back Squat – 3x 3, 3, 3+
2. KB Swing – 4x10
3. Incline DB Bench Press – 4x10
4. Pull Up/BW Row – 4x10
5. Single Arm Suitcase Carry – 3x:40
6. Forward Sled Drag – 12 x 50 Yards w/ 45% of BW

Day 2: S&C (Push/Pull Main, Squat/Hinge Aux + Medium Conditioning)

1. DB Bulgarian Split Squat – 4x10
2. DB RDL – 4x10
3. Barbell Bench Press – 3x 3, 3, 3+
4. T-Bar Row – 3x 5, 5, 5+
5. Sandbag Carry – 3x:40
6. Stairs – x25 Minutes

Day 3: S&C (Hinge Main, Squat, Push, Pull Aux + Easy Conditioning)

1. Goblet Squat - 4x10
2. Conventional Deadlift – 3x 3, 3, 3+
3. Overhead DB Press – 4x10
4. DB Row – 4x10
5. Trap Bar Carry – 3x:40
6. Weight Vest Walk – x25 Minutes

3 Day/Week 3

Day 1: S&C (Squat Main, Hinge/Push/Pull Aux + Easy Conditioning)

1. Barbell Back Squat – 3x 5, 3, 1+
2. KB Swing – 4x12
3. Incline DB Bench Press – 4x12
4. Pull Up/BW Row – 4x12
5. Single Arm Suitcase Carry – 3x45
6. Forward Sled Drag – 12 x 50 Yards w/ 50% of BW

Day 2: S&C (Push/Pull Main, Squat/Hinge Aux + Medium Conditioning)

1. DB Bulgarian Split Squat – 4x12
2. DB RDL – 4x12
3. Barbell Bench Press – 3x 5, 3, 1+
4. T-Bar Row – 4x 5, 5, 5, 5+
5. Sandbag Carry – 3x:45
6. Stairs – x30 Minutes

Day 3: S&C (Hinge Main, Squat, Push, Pull Aux + Easy Conditioning)

1. Goblet Squat -4x12
2. Conventional Deadlift – 3x 5, 3, 1+
3. Overhead DB Press – 4x12
4. DB Row – 4x12
5. Trap Bar Carry – 3x:45
6. Weight Vest Walk – x30 Minutes

3 Day/Week 4 – Deload (Mains should be performed ~50-60% intensity)

Day 1: S&C (Squat Main, Hinge/Push/Pull Aux + Easy Conditioning)

1. Barbell Back Squat – 3x5
2. KB Swing – 3x5
3. Incline DB Bench Press – 3x5
4. Pull Up/BW Row – 3x5
5. Single Arm Suitcase Carry – 3x:30
6. Forward Sled Drag – 12 x 30Yards w/ 35% of BW

Day 2: S&C (Push/Pull Main, Squat/Hinge Aux + Medium Conditioning)

1. Bulgarian Split Squat – 3x5
2. DB RDL – 3x5
3. Barbell Bench Press – 3x5
4. T-Bar Row – 3x5
5. Sandbag Carry – 3x:30
6. Stairs – x20 Minutes

Day 3: S&C (Hinge Main, Squat, Push, Pull Aux + Easy Conditioning)

1. Goblet Squat -3x5
2. Conventional Deadlift – 3x5
3. Overhead DB Press – 3x5
4. DB Row – 3x5
5. Trap Bar Carry – 3x:30
6. Weight Vest Walk – x20 Minutes

3 Day/Week 5

Day 1: S&C (Squat Main, Hinge/Push/Pull Aux + Easy Conditioning)

1. Safety Squat Bar Squat– 3x 5, 5, 5+
2. Hip Thrust– 3x10
3. DB Floor Press – 3x10
4. Lat Pulldown– 3x10
5. Single Arm Bottoms Up KB Carry – 3x:30
6. Backward Sled Drag – 12 x 60 Yards w/ 35% of BW

Day 2: S&C (Push/Pull Main, Squat/Hinge Aux + Medium Conditioning)

1. Hack Squat Machine – 3x10
2. Cable Pull Through – 3x10
3. Incline Bench Press – 3x 5, 5, 5+
4. Bent Over Barbell Row – 3x 8, 8, 8+
5. Odd Object Carry – 3x:30
6. ¼ BW Rucksack Walk – x25 Minutes

Day 3: S&C (Hinge Main, Squat, Push, Pull Aux + Easy Conditioning)

1. Pause Goblet Squat -3x10
2. Deficit Conventional Deadlift – 3x 5, 5, 5+
3. Landmine Press – 3x10
4. Band Pull-a-Part – 3x10
5. Farmers Bar Carry – 3x:30
6. Light Walk/Jog– x25 Minutes

3 Day/Week 6

Day 1: S&C (Squat Main, Hinge/Push/Pull Aux + Easy Conditioning)

1. Safety Squat Bar Squat – 3x 3, 3, 3+
2. Hip Thrust – 4x10
3. DB Floor Press – 4x10
4. Lat Pulldown – 4x10
5. Single Arm Bottoms Up KB Carry – 3x:40
6. Backward Sled Drag – 12 x 60 Yards w/ 45% of BW

Day 2: S&C (Push/Pull Main, Squat/Hinge Aux + Medium Conditioning)

1. Hack Squat – 4x10
2. Cable Pull Through – 4x10
3. Incline Bench Press – 3x 3, 3, 3+
4. Bent Over Row – 3x 5, 5, 5+
5. Odd Object Carry – 3x:40
6. ¼ BW Rucksack Walk – x30 Minutes

Day 3: S&C (Hinge Main, Squat, Push, Pull Aux + Easy Conditioning)

1. Pause Goblet Squat -4x10
2. Deficit Conventional Deadlift – 3x 3, 3, 3+
3. Landmine Press – 4x10
4. Band Pull-a-Part – 4x10
5. Farmers Bar Carry – 3x:40
6. Light Walk/Jog– x30 Minutes

3 Day/Week 7

Day 1: S&C (Squat Main, Hinge/Push/Pull Aux + Easy Conditioning)

1. Safety Squat Bar Squat – 3x 5, 3, 1+
2. Hip Thrust – 4x12
3. DB Floor Press – 4x12
4. Lat Pulldown – 4x12
5. Single Arm Bottoms Up KB Carry – 3x:45
6. Backward Sled Drag – 12 x 50 Yards w/ 50% of BW

Day 2: S&C (Push/Pull Main, Squat/Hinge Aux + Medium Conditioning)

1. Hack Squat – 4x12
2. Cable Pull Through – 4x12
3. Incline Bench Press – 3x 5, 3, 1+
4. Bent Over Row – 4x 5, 5, 5, 5
5. Odd Object Carry – 3x:45
6. ¼ BW Rucksack Walk– x35 Minutes

Day 3: S&C (Hinge Main, Squat, Push, Pull Aux + Easy Conditioning)

1. Pause Goblet Squat -4x12
2. Deficit Conventional Deadlift – 3x 5, 3, 1+
3. Landmine Press – 4x12
4. Band Pull-a-Part – 4x12
5. Farmers Bar Carry – 3x:45
6. Light Walk/Jog– x35 Minutes

3 Day/Week 8 – Deload (Mains should be performed ~50-60% intensity)

Day 1: S&C (Squat Main, Hinge/Push/Pull Aux + Easy Conditioning)

1. Safety Squat Bar Squat – 3x5
2. Hip Thrust – 3x5
3. DB Floor Press – 3x5
4. Lat Pulldown– 3x5
5. Single Arm Bottoms Up Carry – 3x:30
6. Backward Sled Drag – 12 x 30Yards w/ 35% of BW

Day 2: S&C (Push/Pull Main, Squat/Hinge Aux + Medium Conditioning)

1. Hack Squat – 3x5
2. Cable Pull Through– 3x5
3. Incline Bench Press – 3x5
4. Bent Over Row– 3x5
5. Odd Object Carry – 3x:30
6. ¼ BW Rucksack Walk – x20 Minutes

Day 3: S&C (Hinge Main, Squat, Push, Pull Aux + Easy Conditioning)

1. Pause Goblet Squat -3x5
2. Deficit Conventional Deadlift – 3x5
3. Landmine Press – 3x5
4. Band Pull-a-Part – 3x5
5. Farmers Bar Carry – 3x:30
6. Light Walk/Jog – x20 Minutes

3 Day/Week 9

Day 1: S&C (Squat Main, Hinge/Push/Pull Aux + Easy Conditioning)

1. Front Squat – 3x 5, 5, 5+
2. Barbell RDL– 3x10
3. Single Arm KB Overhead Press – 3x10
4. Chin Ups– 3x10
5. KB Front Rack Carry – 3x:30
6. Forward Sled Drag -- 6x60 Yards w/ 35% BW
7. Backward Sled Drag – 6x60 Yards w/ 35% of BW

Day 2: S&C (Push/Pull Main, Squat/Hinge Aux + Medium Conditioning)

1. Landmine Squat – 3x10
2. Single Arm KB Swing – 3x10
3. Barbell Floor Press – 3x 5, 5, 5+
4. Seal Row – 3x 8, 8, 8+
5. KB 2 Hand Carry – 3x:30
6. Medium Intensity Bike Ride – x20 Minutes

Day 3: S&C (Hinge Main, Squat, Push, Pull Aux + Easy Conditioning)

1. Sissy Squat – 3x10
2. Trap Bar Deadlift– 3x 5, 5, 5+
3. Standing Arnold Press – 3x10
4. KB Gorilla Row – 3x10
5. Fat Grip Dumbbell Carry – 3x:30
6. Light Prowler Push – 6x40 Yards

3 Day/Week 10

Day 1: S&C (Squat Main, Hinge/Push/Pull Aux + Easy Conditioning)

1. Front Squat – 3x 3, 3, 3+
2. Barbell RDL – 4x10
3. Single Arm KB Overhead Press – 4x10
4. Chin Ups – 4x10
5. KB Front Rack Carry – 3x:40
6. Forward Sled Drags – 6x60 Yards w/ 45% of BW
7. Backward Sled Drag – 6x60 Yards w/ 45% of BW

Day 2: S&C (Push/Pull Main, Squat/Hinge Aux + Medium Conditioning)

1. Landmine Squat – 4x10
2. Single Arm KB Swing – 4x10
3. Barbell Floor Press – 3x 3, 3, 3+
4. Seal Row – 3x 5, 5, 5+
5. KB 2 Hand Carry – 3x:40
6. Medium Intensity Bike Ride– x25 Minutes

Day 3: S&C (Hinge Main, Squat, Push, Pull Aux + Easy Conditioning)

1. Sissy Squat - 4x10
2. Trap Bar Deadlift – 3x 3, 3, 3+
3. Standing Arnold Press – 4x10
4. KB Gorilla Row – 4x10
5. Fat Grip Dumbbell Carry – 3x:40
6. Light Prowler Push – 8x40 Yards

3 Day/Week 11

Day 1: S&C (Squat Main, Hinge/Push/Pull Aux + Easy Conditioning)

1. Front Squat – 3x 5, 3, 1+
2. Barbell RDL – 4x12
3. Single Arm KB Overhead Press – 4x12
4. Chin Ups – 4x12
5. KB Front Rack Carry – 3x:45
6. Forward Sled Drag – 6x50 Yards w/ 50% BW
7. Backward Sled Drag – 6x50 Yards w/ 50% of BW

Day 2: S&C (Push/Pull Main, Squat/Hinge Aux + Medium Conditioning)

1. Landmine Squat – 4x12
2. Single Arm KB Swing – 4x12
3. Barbell Floor Press – 3x 5, 3, 1+
4. Seal Row – 4x 5, 5, 5, 5+
5. KB 2 Hand Carry – 3x:45
6. Medium Intensity Bike Ride – x30 Minutes

Day 3: S&C (Hinge Main, Squat, Push, Pull Aux + Easy Conditioning)

1. Sissy Squat - 4x12
2. Trap Bar Deadlift – 3x 5, 3, 1+
3. Standing Arnold Press – 4x12
4. KB Gorilla Row – 4x12
5. Fat Grip Dumbbell Carry – 3x:45
6. Light Prowler Push – 10x40 Yards

3 Day/Week 12

You have 3 options here.

Option 1:
Deload the previous 3-week cycle, in similar fashion that you deloaded weeks 1-3 & 5-8's cycle & then start a new cycle the following week. (Week 13)

Option 2:
If you're feeling good, go ahead & program another 3-week cycle using the outline exemplified in weeks 1-11.

Option 3:
If you have any Personal Record (PR) Goals, whether they be 1RM's, Rep Maxes, or Conditioning Challenges, feel free to use this week to test yourself. After a testing week, you may deload, start a new 3-week cycle, or do what you wish with your training.

12-Week/3-Day Minimalist Template

The Minimalist option is great option for those with minimal time, equipment, etc. You need nothing more than your body & a single Kettlebell, Dumbbell, Rock, etc. Don't worry too much about the Main/Aux concepts here. Use what you have.

You'll notice I've broken the set & rep *rules* to accommodate for the lack of resistance/variation.

3 Day Minimalist/Week 1

Day 1: Strength & Conditioning

1. KB Goblet Squat – 3x10
2. KB Swing – 3x10
3. Bottoms Up KB Press – 3x10
4. KB 1 Arm Row – 3x10
5. KB Goblet Carry – 3x :30
6. 1 Mile Walk

Day 3: Strength & Conditioning

1. KB Bulgarian Split Squat – 3x10 Ea. Leg
2. KB 'Belly Hinge' – 3x10 Ea. Leg
3. Push Up – 3x10
4. Bodyweight Row – 3x10
5. Single Arm KB Carry – 3x :30
6. Hill Sprints – 10x 30 yards

Day 5: Strength & Conditioning

1. Bodyweight Squat – 3x25
2. KB RDL – 3x10
3. KB Incline Press – 3x10
4. KB Upright Row – 3x10
5. KB Bottoms Up Carry – 3x :30
6. Stadium Steps – 20 Minutes

3 Day Minimalist/Week 2

Day 1: Strength & Conditioning

1. KB Goblet Squat – 4x10
2. KB Swing – 4x10
3. Bottoms Up KB Press – 4x10
4. KB 1 Arm Row – 4x10
5. KB Goblet Carry – 3x :40
6. 1.5 Mile Walk

Day 3: Strength & Conditioning

1. KB Bulgarian Split Squat – 4x10 Ea. Leg
2. KB 'Belly Hinge' – 4x10 Ea. Leg
3. Push Up – 4x10
4. Bodyweight Row – 4x10
5. Single Arm KB Carry – 3x :40
6. Hill Sprints – 12x 30 yards

Day 5: Strength & Conditioning

1. Bodyweight Squat – 4x25
2. KB RDL – 4x10
3. KB Incline Press – 4x10
4. KB Upright Row – 4x10
5. KB Bottoms Up Carry – 3x :40
6. Stadium Steps – 25 Minutes

3 Day Minimalist/Week 3

Day 1: Strength & Conditioning

1. KB Goblet Squat – 4x12
2. KB Swing – 4x12
3. Bottoms Up KB Press – 4x12
4. KB 1 Arm Row – 4x12
5. KB Goblet Carry – 3x :45
6. 2 Mile Walk

Day 3: Strength & Conditioning

1. KB Bulgarian Split Squat – 4x12 Ea. Leg
2. KB 'Belly Hinge' – 4x12 Ea. Leg
3. Push Up – 4x12
4. Bodyweight Row – 4x12
5. Single Arm KB Carry – 3x:45
6. Hill Sprints – 15x 30 yards

Day 5: Strength & Conditioning

1. Bodyweight Squat – 5x25
2. KB RDL – 4x12
3. KB Incline Press – 4x12
4. KB Upright Row – 4x12
5. KB Bottoms Up Carry – 3x:45
6. Stadium Steps – 30 Minutes

3 Day Minimalist/Week 4 – Deload Week

Day 1: Strength & Conditioning

1. KB Goblet Squat – 2x10
2. KB Swing – 2x10
3. Bottoms Up KB Press – 2x10
4. KB 1 Arm Row – 2x10
5. KB Goblet Carry – 2x :30
6. 1 Mile Walk

Day 3: Strength & Conditioning

1. KB Bulgarian Split Squat – 3x5 Ea. Leg
2. KB 'Belly Hinge' – 2x10 Ea. Leg
3. Push Up – 2x10
4. Bodyweight Row – 2x10
5. Single Arm KB Carry – 3x :30
6. Hill Sprints – 8x 30 yards

Day 5: Strength & Conditioning

1. Bodyweight Squat – 2x25
2. KB RDL – 2x10
3. KB Incline Press – 2x10
4. KB Upright Row – 2x10
5. KB Bottoms Up Carry – 2x:30
6. Stadium Steps – 20 Minutes

3 Day Minimalist/Week 5

Day 1: Strength & Conditioning

1. KB Goblet Squat w/ 2 Sec. Pause in Bottom – 3x10
2. KB Swing – 4x10
3. Bottoms Up KB Press, 3 Sec. Up, 3 Sec. Down Tempo – 3x10
4. KB 1 Arm Row – 4x10
5. KB Goblet Carry – 4x :35
6. KB Carry – 20 minutes

Day 3: Strength & Conditioning

1. KB Bulgarian Split Squat w/ 2 Sec. Pause in Bottom – 3x10 Ea. Leg
2. Single Leg KB RDL – 3x10
3. Push Up, 3 Sec. Down, 3 Sec. Up Tempo – 3x10
4. Bodyweight Row – 4x10
5. Single Arm KB Carry – 3x :35
6. Sprints – 10x 40 yards

Day 5: Strength & Conditioning

1. 1 ½ Rep Bodyweight Squat – 3x20
2. KB Deadlift – 3x25
3. Seated KB Overhead Press – 3x10
4. Chin Up – 3x10
5. KB Bottoms Up Carry – 3x:35
6. Jog – 20 Minutes

3 Day Minimalist/Week 6

Day 1: Strength & Conditioning

1. KB Goblet Squat w/ 2 Sec. Pause in Bottom – 4x10
2. KB Swing – 4x12
3. Bottoms Up KB Press, 3 Sec. Up, 3 Sec. Down Tempo – 4x10
4. KB 1 Arm Row – 4x12
5. KB Goblet Carry – 4x :40
6. KB Carry – 25 minutes

Day 3: Strength & Conditioning

1. KB Bulgarian Split Squat w/ 2 Sec. Pause in Bottom – 4x10 Ea. Leg
2. KB 'Belly Hinge' – 4x12
3. Push Up, 3 Sec. Down, 3 Sec. Up Tempo – 4x10
4. Bodyweight Row – 4x12
5. Single Arm KB Carry – 3x :40
6. Sprints – 12x 30 yards

Day 5: Strength & Conditioning

1. 1 ½ Rep Bodyweight Squat – 3x25
2. KB Deadlift – 4x25
3. Seated KB Overhead Press – 4x10
4. Chin Up – 4x10
5. KB Bottoms Up Carry – 3x:40
6. Jog – 25 Minutes

3 Day Minimalist/Week 7

Day 1: Strength & Conditioning

1. KB Goblet Squat w/ 2 Sec. Pause in Bottom – 4x12
2. KB Swing – 6x10
3. Bottoms Up KB Press, 3 Sec. Up, 3 Sec. Down Tempo – 4x12
4. KB 1 Arm Row – 5x12
5. KB Goblet Carry – 4x :45
6. KB Carry – 20 minutes

Day 3: Strength & Conditioning

1. KB Bulgarian Split Squat w/ 2 Sec. Pause in Bottom – 5x12 Ea. Leg
2. KB 'Belly Hinge' – 5x12
3. Push Up, 3 Sec. Down, 3 Sec. Up Tempo – 4x12
4. Bodyweight Row – 5x12
5. Single Arm KB Carry – 3x :45
6. Sprints – 15x 30 yards

Day 5: Strength & Conditioning

1. 1 ½ Rep Bodyweight Squat – 3x30
2. KB Deadlift – 5x25
3. Seated KB Overhead Press – 4x12
4. Chin Up – 5x10
5. KB Bottoms Up Carry – 3x:45
6. Jog – 30 Minutes

3 Day Minimalist/Week 8 – Deload Week

Day 1: Strength & Conditioning

1. KB Goblet Squat w/ 2 Sec. Pause in Bottom – 2x10
2. KB Swing – 2x10
3. Bottoms Up KB Press, 3 Sec. Up, 3 Sec. Down Tempo – 2x10
4. KB 1 Arm Row – 2x10
5. KB Goblet Carry – 3x :35
6. KB Carry – 20 minutes

Day 3: Strength & Conditioning

1. KB Bulgarian Split Squat w/ 2 Sec. Pause in Bottom – 2x10 Ea. Leg
2. KB 'Belly Hinge' – 3x10 Ea. Leg
3. Push Up, 3 Sec. Down, 3 Sec. Up Tempo – 2x10
4. Bodyweight Row – 2x10
5. Single Arm KB Carry – 3x :35
6. Sprints – 8x 40 yards

Day 5: Strength & Conditioning

1. 1 ½ Rep Bodyweight Squat – 2x20
2. KB Deadlift – 2x25
3. Seated KB Overhead Press – 2x10
4. Chin Up – 2x10
5. KB Bottoms Up Carry – 3x:35
6. Jog – 20 Minutes

3 Day Minimalist/Week 9

Day 1: Strength & Conditioning

1. KB Goblet Squat 3 sec. Down, 3 Sec. Up – 3x10
2. KB Swing – 4x12
3. Bottoms Up KB Press 3 Sec. Hold in Bottom – 3x10
4. KB Gorilla Row – 3x10 Ea. Arm
5. KB Goblet Carry – 4x :40
6. ¼ BW Pound Backpack Walk – 20 minutes

Day 3: Strength & Conditioning

1. Bottoms Up KB Goblet Squat, 3 Sec. Down, 1 Sec. Up – 3x10
2. Single Leg KB RDL – 4x10 Ea. Leg
3. Push Up, 3 Sec. Down, 3 Sec. Up Tempo – 3x10
4. Pull Up – 3x10
5. Single Arm KB Carry – 4x :40
6. Sprints – 10x 50 yards

Day 5: Strength & Conditioning

1. Bodyweight Sissy Squat – 3x10
2. Sumo Stance KB Deadlift – 3x10
3. Standing Bottoms Up KB Press – 3x10
4. KB Upright Row – 3x10
5. KB Bottoms Up Carry – 4x :40
6. Trail Run – 20 Minutes

3 Day Minimalist/Week 10

Day 1: Strength & Conditioning

1. KB Goblet Squat 3 sec. Down, 3 Sec. Up – 4x10
2. KB Swing – 4x15
3. Bottoms Up KB Press 3 Sec. Hold in Bottom – 4x10
4. KB Gorilla Row – 4x10 Ea. Arm
5. KB Goblet Carry – 4x :45
6. ¼ BW Pound Backpack Walk – 30 minutes

Day 3: Strength & Conditioning

1. Bottoms Up KB Goblet Squat, 3 Sec. Down, 1 Sec. Up – 4x10
2. Single Leg KB RDL – 4x12 Ea. Leg
3. Push Up, 3 Sec. Down, 3 Sec. Up Tempo – 5x10
4. Pull Up – 4x12
5. Single Arm KB Carry – 4x :50
6. Sprints – 15x 50 yards

Day 5: Strength & Conditioning

1. Bodyweight Sissy Squat – 3x20
2. Sumo Stance KB Deadlift – 3x20
3. Standing Bottoms Up KB Press – 3x20
4. KB Upright Row – 3x20
5. KB Bottoms Up Carry – 4x :50
6. Trail Run – 30 Minutes

3 Day Minimalist/Week 11

Day 1: Strength & Conditioning

1. KB Goblet Squat 3 sec. Down, 3 Sec. Up – 4x12
2. KB Swing – 5x12
3. Bottoms Up KB Press 3 Sec. Hold in Bottom – 4x12
4. KB Gorilla Row – 4x12 Ea. Arm
5. KB Goblet Carry – 4x :50
6. ¼ BW Pound Backpack Walk – 30 minutes

Day 3: Strength & Conditioning

1. Bottoms Up KB Goblet Squat, 3 Sec. Down, 1 Sec. Up – 5x10
2. Single Leg KB RDL – 4x12 Ea. Leg
3. Push Up, 3 Sec. Down, 3 Sec. Up Tempo – 4x10
4. Pull Up – 4x10
5. Single Arm KB Carry – 4x :45
6. Sprints – 12x 50 yards

Day 5: Strength & Conditioning

1. Bodyweight Sissy Squat – 3x15
2. Sumo Stance KB Deadlift – 3x15
3. Standing Bottoms Up KB Press – 3x15
4. KB Upright Row – 3x15
5. KB Bottoms Up Carry – 4x :45
6. Trail Run – 25 Minutes

3 Day Minimalist/Week 12

You have 3 options here.

Option 1:
Deload the previous 3-week cycle, in similar fashion that you deloaded weeks 1-3 & 5-8's cycle & then start a new cycle the following week. (Week 13)

Option 2:
If you're feeling good, go ahead & program another 3-week cycle using the outline exemplified in weeks 1-11.

Option 3:
If you have any Personal Record (PR) Goals, whether they be 1RM's, Rep Maxes, or Conditioning Challenges, feel free to use this week to test yourself. After a testing week, you may deload, start a new 3-week cycle, or do what you wish with your training.

*Obviously with the minimalist templates, it will be wise to *break the rules* depending on your strength levels/how much weight/equipment you have access to. Do not undervalue calisthenics & the art of making light weights, heavy.

Get creative and make the most out of what you have access to. It will serve you far better than complaining about what you don't have or can't do 100 out of 100 times.

Sources:

Easter, Michael. *The Comfort Crisis: Embrace Discomfort to Reclaim Your Wild, Happy, Healthy Self*. Rodale Books, 2021.

Jamieson, Joel. *Ultimate MMA Conditioning*. Performance Sports Inc., 2009.

John, Dan. *Attempts* On Target Publications 2020

Wendler, Jim. *5/3/1: The Simplest and Most Effective Training System to Increase Raw Strength.* Jim Wendler LLC, 2011.

Wendler, Jim. *5/3/1 Forever: Simple and Effective Programming for Size, Speed, and Strength.* Jim Wendler LLC, 2017.

Tsatouline, Pavel. *Simple And Sinister.* StrongFirst, Inc.; 2nd edition 2019

Yellowhousedesign. "Joe D's 'Limber 11' (Flexibility Routine)." *Official Website of Joe DeFranco & DeFranco's Gym!*, 4 July 2015, https://www.defrancostraining.com/joe-ds-qlimber-11q-flexibility-routine/.

Yellowhousedesign. "Westside for Skinny Bastards, Part III." *Official Website of Joe DeFranco & DeFranco's Gym!*, 3 July 2015, https://www.defrancostraining.com/westside-for-skinny-bastards-part3/.

Notes:

Notes:

Notes:

Notes:

About The Author

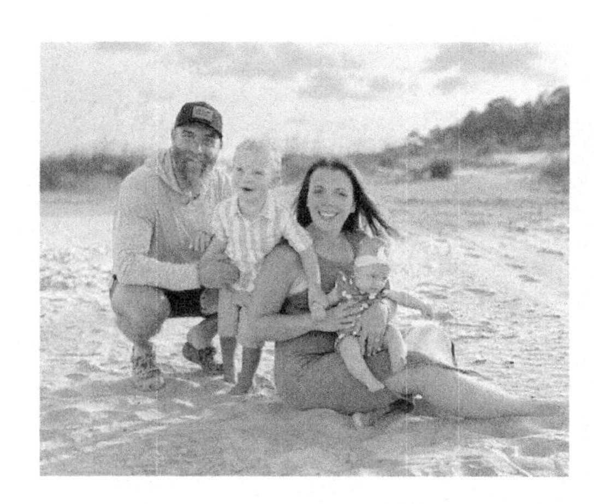

Ray Zingler, CPPS

Ray is a Strength Coach, Entrepreneur, & Consultant.

He is the Owner of Zingler Strength & Conditioning, LLC., an industry leader in performance training for athletes, busy professionals, and military personnel.

Ray is recognized as a Certified Physical Preparation Specialist and has been serving the Metro Atlanta, Georgia area since 2009. His blue collar, nothing fancy, just consistency and hard work approach to research based training has allowed him to serve thousands of clients.

In addition to his brick and mortar gym, Ray consults current and prospective gym owners on business structure and implementation.

Beyond mentoring strength professionals, Ray consults with high school sport and strength coaches, aiding in the development of program structure and design.

Finally, Ray does contract work within local high schools and club sport organizations, implementing S&C programs within the team settings of a variety of sports.

Ray and his Wife Courtney own and operate Zingler Strength & Conditioning in Marietta, GA and reside in Woodstock, GA with their son Raymond Mac, daughter Jolene, and a property full of dogs, cats, and chickens.

Ray is an avid reader, writer, working dog enthusiast, and deer hunter. Most importantly he is an unashamed blood bought follower of Jesus Christ.

Made in the USA
Las Vegas, NV
14 April 2024